Clinical Research Methodology and Evidence-based Medicine: The Basics

Clinical Research Methodology and Evidence-based Medicine: The Basics

Ajit N. Babu, MBBS, MPH, FACP
Professor of Medicine
Director, Centre for Digital Health (CDH)
Chairman, Institute of Medical Informatics and
Multimedia Education (IMIME)
Amrita Institute of Medical Sciences
Cochin, Kerala, INDIA
and
Clinical Associate Professor of Medicine,
Saint Louis University
Staff Physician, St. Louis VA Medical Center,
St. Louis, MO, USA

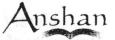

Anshan Limited, (UK)

Anshan Limited
6 Newlands Road
Tunbride Wells
Kent TN4 9AT, UK
Tel/Fax: +44(0) 1892 557767
e-mail: infor@anshan.co.uk
website: www.anshan.co.uk

© 2008 BI Publications Pvt Ltd
Published 2008

British Library Cataloguing in Publication Data
A catalogue record for this book is available from the British Library.

Not for sale in India, Pakistan, Nepal, Sri Lanka and Bangladesh

ISBN: 978-1-905740-90-1

This edition is co-published by B.I. Publication Pvt. Ltd., New Delhi, India and Anshan Limited, Kent, UK, and printed at Saurabh Printers Pvt. Ltd., Noida, India.

Preface

Is there a cure for cancer? Can we find an effective treatment for Alzheimer's? Are there ways to eliminate coronary artery disease? The answers to these and countless other questions of grave importance to humanity depend on effective and energetic medical research.

Around the world, there are increasing requirements for medical trainees to understand research methodology and to do at least one research project as a mandatory part of their training. In many Western countries, academic advancement for medical faculty is contingent upon research productivity. Unfortunately, only a small fraction of the path-breaking discoveries in medicine have originated in the developing world. The paucity of infrastructure and funding is clearly responsible to a degree. But, it is also evident that a lack of appreciation of the importance of research and the absence of proper training have contributed to this troubling inadequacy.

A related concept, which is also being discussed and debated in forums around the globe, is that of Evidence-based Medicine (EBM), which presents systematic guidance for frontline clinicians in applying research principles and findings to their patient care.

Though these topics are interconnected in many ways, there is a scarcity of material that concurrently provides the novice a basic and affordable introduction to these two subjects. This book is meant to serve as a primer for beginners who have had an interest, or perhaps even a need, to learn more about medical research methodology and Evidence-based Medicine. After all, the future belongs to them.

Ajit N. Babu

Acknowledgements

This book would not have been possible without the expertise brought to bear by the contributors to this work - Dr. Steven Kymes, Dr. S. N. Sarbadhikari, Ms. Vasumathi Sriganesh, Dr. James Stahl and Mr. R. Vinaitheerthan. I am truly grateful to them for the diligence of their efforts and the elegance of their writing. Furthermore, I wish to record my appreciation for the exceptional support provided by the team from BI Publishers - Mr. Y. R. Chadha and Dr. B. C. Sharma for their editorial oversight, and Mr. Vinod K.V., Manager, Kochi office, whose persistence was instrumental in my attempting this work in the first place.

On a broader level, I also express my gratitude to the Amrita Institute of Medical Sciences, Kochi for providing me with an outstanding professional environment conducive to academic research and scholarship of an international standard.

Most of all, I acknowledge with deepest affection my wife Madhu and children Giridhar and Gauri who grumbled at my absences from family life while working on this manuscript, yet cheerfully welcomed me to the dinner table on the rare occasions when I made it there on time...!

Ajit N. Babu
Kochi, India

Contributors

Primary Author

Ajit N. Babu, MBBS, MPH, FACP, Professor of Medicine, Director, Centre for Digital Health (CDH); Chairman, Institute of Medical Informatics and Multimedia Education (IMIME), Amrita Institute of Medical Sciences, Cochin, Kerala, INDIA and Clinical Associate Professor of Medicine, Saint Louis University; Staff Physician, St. Louis VA Medical Center, St. Louis, MO, USA

Contributors

Steven M. Kymes, PhD, MHA., Research Assistant Professor, Washington University School of Medicine, Department of Ophthalmology and Visual Sciences, Senior Research Fellow Washington University Center for Health Policy, St. Louis, MO, USA

S. N. Sarbadhikari, MBBS, PhD, Associate Professor of Biomedical Engineering, TIFAC-CORE in Biomedical Technology, Amrita Vishwa Vidyapeetham, Amritapuri, Kerala, INDIA and Centre for Digital Health (CDH), Amrita Institute of Medical Sciences, Cochin, Kerala, INDIA

Vasumathi Sriganesh, BSc, MLIS, Director, QMed Services, Mumbai, Maharashtra, INDIA

James Stahl, MD, CM, MPH, Senior Scientist, Massachusetts General Hospital–Institute for Technology Assessment, Assistant Professor of Medicine, Harvard Medical School, Boston, MA, USA

R. Vinaitheerthan, MSc, MCA, Lecturer, Biostatistics, Centre for Digital Health (CDH), Amrita Institute of Medical Sciences, Cochin, Kerala, INDIA

Contents

1. Introduction   1
    Ajit N. Babu

2. Ethics in Healthcare   7
    Ajit N. Babu

3. Introduction to Biostatistics   28
    R. Vinaitheerthan and Ajit N. Babu

4. Research Methodology   61
    Ajit N. Babu

5. An Introduction to Medical Decision-making   72
    James Stahl

6. Sources of Evidence and How to Use Them   83
    Vasumathi Sriganesh

7. An Overview of Evidence-based Medicine
    (EBM) and Critical Appraisal   93
    Ajit N. Babu

8. EBM and Therapy   104
    Ajit N. Babu

9. EBM and Diagnosis   111
    Steven Kymes

10. EBM and Prognosis   134
    Ajit N. Babu

x Contents

11. EBM and Economic Analysis   141
    Steven Kymes

12. Translating EBM into Practice   159
    Ajit N. Babu

13. Evidence-based Medicine and Medical Informatics:
    The Role of Clinical Decision Support
    Systems (CDSS)   166
    S.N. Sarbadhikari

Index   179

Introduction

Ajit N. Babu

Research methodology can be thought of as the discipline concerned with the scientific conception, design, implementation and analysis of research. *Evidence-based Medicine (EBM)* is an approach for *evaluating and applying* medical knowledge, particularly that derived from original research, in the care of individual patients. Since these two entities really form a continuum, this book has combined them to give the reader a sound introduction to these related subjects.

The practice and teaching of medicine is a vital endeavor. Without being trite, it can truly be said that lives depend on it. Medical practitioners over the ages have surrounded themselves with an aura of sagacity, evoking a mixture of respect, awe and perhaps envy. The truth of the matter though is that there are vast provinces of medical care that remain poorly defined or frankly unknown. Medicine has traditionally not dealt well with uncertainty, at times skirting around this difficult terrain with more bluff and bluster than substance. The ideal way of tackling ignorance is to convert the unknown to the known by careful study and thoughtful analysis. Important medical questions should be answered through meticulous research that is designed to specifically study the issue. From an individual clinician's perspective, the most valid research not only has strong study design, but is also conducted with a patient population and clinical environment similar to those encountered by the clinician. Properly designed and conducted research is the foundation of credible medical knowledge. One of the key elements of a successful research project is proper statistical evaluation and design such that the methodology for the project is likely to yield valid answers to the questions being posed. The field of statistics owes a great deal to Karl Pearson, a Professor of Mathematics at University College, London who is widely regarded as one of the founders of modern statistics. One of his pupils, Major Greenwood, is credited with being the first medical statistician as he argued forcefully for the use of statistical methods in medicine to make it more scientific. Greenwood joined the Medical Research Council in the United Kingdom in 1920. This event had far reaching consequences, as his successors conducted the first randomized controlled clinical trial to address an important clinical question – the value of streptomycin added to bed rest in the treatment of TB compared to bed rest alone. Streptomycin was found to be superior, and with the wisdom of hindsight, we know that this is indeed the case.[1]

From these early beginnings, medical research has evolved into an increasingly sophisticated discipline that uses advanced theories of research design, statistics and, of late, informatics.

A fundamental change that has also occurred over the last few decades in the interface of medical research and the practicing profession is the increasing expectation from both society and the medical community that medical practitioners be familiar not only with prescribing medications or ordering tests, but also the scientific basis on which management decisions are made. The tidal wave of information that the Internet has unleashed has opened up new sources and modalities of knowledge acquisition and dissemination. These days, it is common in societies around the world to have patients and their relatives going to meet the doctor clutching a sheaf of printouts relating to the patients' medical condition (real or imagined) from "The Net". This phenomenon raises an important question: How does one decide if the information one is presented or obtains is valid? In this context, the word "valid" relates to authenticity, truthfulness and scientific accuracy.

Information coming from trusted medical sources like a major journal or the website of an established medical society may be considered authentic and most likely truthful. However, there have been well-publicized instances of academic fraud, underlining the fact that we should not take anything for granted. The final part relating to scientific accuracy is more complex. Even two intelligent and knowledgeable medical professionals could interpret a given piece of information in different ways, or come to divergent conclusions from the same set of research results. One of the difficulties in medical research is the inherent variation among human beings. The whole spectrum of physiological states that are compatible with wellness or disease are sometimes difficult to confirm with certainty much less measure with accuracy.

Another element of applied informatics that is having a greater impact on medical practice is the electronic medical record (EMR) system. Traditionally, medical record keeping has been on paper, and this continues to be the practice in many hospitals and clinics around the world. There has been increasing recognition that electronic records can allow better storage, retrieval and analysis of medical information. Electronic systems initially started with demographic and financial information. It later started to include laboratory data. Recent entrants have been electronic orders, notes and digital images that are stored on a Picture Archiving and Communication System (PACS). These developments have important implications not only for clinical practice but also for research because of the dynamic possibilities that are brought about to improve access to information at what is called "the point of care" – the location in space and time where a given episode of healthcare is being delivered. The available information can be passive - where you get what you ask for (e.g., a literature search on the Internet) or active - wherein the computer system gives advice, recommendations or hints based on its knowledge base to assist the clinician in making a management decision even without the clinical asking for help. The latter form of information delivery is embodied in computerized Clinical Decision Support Systems (CDSS) that work best when seamlessly interfaced with an EMR system. CDSS can track multiple patient characteristics and potentially give alerts or prompts in meaningful circumstances without a direct request from the user. For example, if a physician writes an order for aspirin for a patient who is documented in the EMR to have an allergy to aspirin, the EMR CDSS will then generate an alert (typically as a pop-up box) pointing this out and asking for a justification before it accepts the physician's order. There are also stand-alone CDSS programs that function more in the manner of an interactive textbook, responding to queries posed by the user – such as a listing of signs and symptoms with pertinent patient demographic information – by giving a list of potential diagnoses.

The concept of EBM applies many of the principles and technologies discussed above. In the last decade and a half, EBM has become an increasingly popular catchword, and there has been an explosion of information about the methodology for critical appraisal that is the heart of EBM. It is true, but not often highlighted, that many of the fundamentals of EBM are drawn from the field of clinical epidemiology. The real success of the EBM movement lies in the fact that key concepts once regarded by frontline clinicians as the obscure mutterings of a rather musty scientific discipline have become widely accepted and *familiar* to even non-academic clinicians and healthcare professionals. These days, it is rare to find a conference or a journal which does not make at least passing reference to "evidence-based something-or-the-other". EBM essentially has given a set of guidelines and concept applications that can be used to evaluate medical literature even by non-experts. A series of publications spanning well over a decade in the *Journal of the American Medical Association (JAMA)* have examined the EBM approach to take for a variety of article types – those dealing with therapy, diagnosis, harm, prognosis and so on.

Unfortunately, despite these progressive developments, many physicians, even those who are sub-specialists or in academia, have only a sketchy understanding of research methodology and evaluation or of EBM. This book is a modest attempt to help bridge the gap, and is directed towards the novice. The contributors to this work are all experts drawn from India and the United States, who have years of experience in evaluating, applying and using the concepts and methods they have written about. Each of the elements discussed above have been targeted for inclusion in one or more chapters so that the reader gets a multifaceted view of research, EBM and interconnected areas. The one exception is EMR – a detailed exposition and exploration of the topic is beyond the scope of this book, and probably would be of marginal interest to young trainees, junior clinicians and other healthcare professionals - the intended readership for this work.

The chapters in this book are meant to be self-supporting and can be read out of sequence to a fair extent; however, it is probable that the greatest utility from the book would be derived in reading it cover to cover. A quick recounting of the content and sequence of the remaining chapters of this book would seem to be in order. The second chapter gives an overview of healthcare ethics. Chapter 3 provides an introduction to biostatistics, with a focus on approaches most relevant to clinical research and EBM. This is followed by the fourth chapter that takes a broad look at research methodology. The fifth chapter reviews basic principles and techniques of medical decision-making. Chapter 6 presents a concise overview of Internet resources for medical professionals. The seventh chapter commences the section of the book dealing with EBM by giving an overview followed by four more chapters on therapy, diagnosis, prognosis and economic analysis, respectively. The last has been included, since a basic understanding of healthcare economics and its impact on how healthcare systems function is crucial for the well-informed medical practitioner, and it is an area that is particularly neglected in medical education, especially in India and other developing countries. Chapter 12 presents some practical strategies for using these principles in real-world settings. The book concludes with Chapter 13, which details how CDSS applications of medical informatics can assist in the practice of EBM.

Each chapter gives suggested resources for further reading at the end that can supplement and expand on the topic covered. Keep in mind that most of these materials have their origin in North America and Europe – the relevance of their recommendations must be carefully weighed in the context of your own environment, circumstances and resources.

The book summary in the preceding paragraphs may give the impression that a vast volume of material is being covered – it is not. There are fairly detailed reviews of core subjects at a level suitable for a beginner accompanied by broad overviews of related topics. Interested readers would be well advised to consult more detailed textbooks for greater insight.

Knowledge of research methodology, EBM and related advances in informatics will be of value to any healthcare professional. However, it must also be stated plainly that technologies like the EMR have a long way to go before these are suitable for widespread use. EBM also has its own fallacies and foibles. Being a relatively new school of thought, there are bugs that are still being worked out. Unfortunately, there are some who are so passionate about EBM that they lose all perspective and common sense and try to fit everything in an EBM box, throwing out with the trash whatever does not. There are others who are vehemently opposed to EBM, regarding the whole exercise with scorn and suspicion. Like zealots of any ilk, individuals in either of these camps can be rather volatile, so tread carefully around them as you commence your journey of exploration...!

Reference

1. Chen TT. History of statistical thinking in medicine. In: Lu Y, Fang JQ, editors. *Advanced Medical Statistics.* Singapore: World Scientific Publishing Co; 2003:9-14.

Recommended Resources

1. Clinicians for the Restoration of Autonomous Practice Writing Group. EBM: unmasking the ugly truth. BMJ. 2002; 325:1496-1498.

2. Evidence-based Medicine Working Group. Evidence-based medicine: a new approach to teaching the practice of medicine. *JAMA.* 1992;268:2420-2425.

3. Fletcher RH, Fletcher SW, Wagner EH. *Clinical Epidemiology: The Essentials.* 3rd ed. Baltimore, Maryland: Williams & Wilkins; 1996.

4. Guyatt GH, Rennie D. Users' guides to the medical literature. *JAMA.* 1993;270:2096-2097.

5. Oxman AD, Sackett DL, Guyatt GH, for the Evidence-Based Medicine Working Group. Users' guides to the medical literature, I: how to get started. *JAMA.* 1993;270:2093-2095.

6. Sackett DL, Haynes RB, Guyatt GH, Tugwell P. *Clinical Epidemiology: A Basic Science for Clinical Medicine.* 2nd ed. Boston, Mass: Little Brown & Co Inc; 1991:145-148.

7. Sackett DL, Straus SE, Richardson WS, et al. *Evidence-based Medicine: How to Practice and Teach EBM.* Toronto, Ontario: Churchill Livingstone; 1998.

8. Centre for Health Evidence User's Guide to Evidence-based Practice at: *http://www.cche.net/usersguides/main.asp*

9. JAMA Users' Guides to the Medical Literature at: *http://ugi.usersguides.org/usersguides/hg/hh_start.asp.*

2

Ethics in Healthcare

Ajit N. Babu

- Introduction

- Ethical Conduct of
  Research

- The Declaration of
  Helsinki

- The Principles of Good
  Clinical Practice (GCP)

- Ethics in Medical Writing

- COPE guidelines

- The Medical Industry and
  Healthcare Providers—
  Where Is the Ethical
  Meeting Ground?

- Warning Signs of an
  Unethical Milieu

- Ethics in Clinical Practice

Introduction

Medicine is a field with unique ethical concepts. Medicine cannot be thought of as a business, though by necessity many of its actions, such as the running of a clinic or hospital, may need to be regulated by business principles for the sake of fiscal survival. However, ethical tenets that are considered satisfactory and even appropriate in a business setting may be unacceptable in Medicine. While there are broad principles of medical ethics that are common across cultures, there are differences as well. For instance, in Asia there is a component of paternalistic practice on the part of the physician that is regarded as acceptable and indeed desirable by patients and their families. In a Western context, such behavior would be deemed inappropriate and instead a participatory format where both the healthcare team and the patient are equals in the relationship is the seen as the most equitable approach.

Ethical Conduct of Research

In clinical research, there are special obligations brought upon the investigators to protect human subjects. In the West, there are increasingly stringent rules and regulations promulgated by governmental oversight entities to ensure the safety of human subjects after a variety of scandals and ethical improprieties came to light. The unfortunate consequence of this changing environment has been the hampering of creativity and intellectual growth, since research has become such a complex enterprise that an unfunded young researcher faces a daunting task in executing a successful project – so much so that many researchers give up the attempt.

Any research endeavor, no matter how attractive purely from a study design standpoint, is unworthy of consideration or acceptance if it is ethically compromised. The classic (and horrifying) examples that are often quoted of "science" run amok are that of the Tuskeegee study and the experiments by Nazi doctors on prisoners of war.

The Tuskeegee study was funded by the US government in the early 1930's to determine the effects of untreated syphilis on black American males. In pursuit of this goal, a cohort of patients who were evaluated for this disorder in government clinics in the poor rural area of Tuskeegee, Alabama were followed over time. In a manner that would be unthinkable today, these unwitting patients deliberately had penicillin, which became available a decade later (at that time literally a wonder drug that was dramatically effective against syphilis), withheld so that they could suffer from the full ravages of the disease unfettered by the benefits of medication! A newspaper investigative report in 1972 brought this infamy to light, and led to a public outcry. The study was stopped, with the subjects and affected family members being offered free lifelong treatment. As a result, there were sweeping changes in the oversight process of American research after the National Research Act of 1974 that was followed by publication of an official document, called the Belmont Report, which still guides the ethical conduct of American research. Many other nations have adopted these, or other similar principles. Sadly, there remains a deep mistrust of medical research among some black Americans that hinders their full participation in research even today, limiting our understanding in some instances of the effects of new therapies in this community.

The Belmont Report highlighted three fundamental principles, which are very similar to that generally accepted as key elements (Fig. 2.1) of Western medical ethics – autonomy, beneficence and justice:

- **Respect for persons**–includes recognition of autonomy and the provision of additional protections and care to those who by virtue of infirmity or socio-economic circumstances are vulnerable to external pressure or inducements.

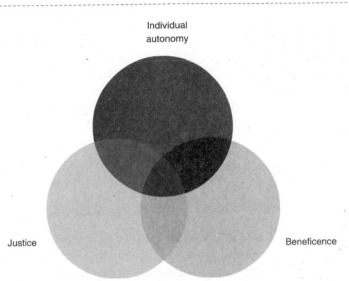

Fig. 2.1. Basic elements of medical ethics

- **Beneficence**–the concept of going beyond the minimum required to ensure the well-being of subjects.

- **Justice**–the need for fairness in the distribution of the benefits and risks of research, in the context of benefits to individuals and society at large.

The end of World War II brought to light the atrocities committed by the Nazis on concentration camp inmates in the name of science. For instance, prisoners were immersed in ice-cold water even to the point of death to "learn" about the possible effects of cold-water immersion on Nazi aviators who may be shot down over the ocean. At the epoch making trials at Nuremberg in 1946, a number of Nazi physicians were in the dock. Though they tried to defend themselves by stating they were merely carrying out orders, the culpability of these physicians in these heinous acts was readily evident, and their actions remain an indelible defilement of the medical profession and humanity at large. The trials led to the promulgation of the Nuremberg Code that was a watershed in enhancing the ethical conduct of research. Important concepts like informed consent, avoidance of unwarranted risk to subjects and scientific validity of the research hypothesis were brought forth and went on to form the cornerstones of modern ethical processes in research.

The Declaration of Helsinki

The 1964 meeting of the World Medical Association (WMA) at Helsinki, Finland resulted in the Declaration of Helsinki that outlined cardinal principles in medical ethics and serves as the gold standard worldwide. Recently, in 2000, there were some revisions to the guidelines which led to international expressions of concern about the modifications weakening oversight requirements such that placebo trials were proposed to be ethically appropriate, even when more effective therapies were available.

The Principles of Good Clinical Practice (GCP)

The latter half of the 20th century saw acceleration in the generation of rules, regulations and laws for evaluating new therapeutic products. Although various regulatory systems were based on the same core obligations to evaluate quality, safety and efficacy, the actual technical requirements had diverged over time to an enormous degree leading to duplication of efforts and organizational inefficiency. At the same time, there was increasing public pressure to expediently bring to market potentially efficacious remedies. There was growing realization that it was important to have an independent evaluation of medicinal products before they are allowed in the market and that it was essential to have collaboration between major stakeholders to allow this to happen with the greatest efficiency and cost-effectiveness.

The International Conference on Harmonization of Technical Requirements for Registration of Pharmaceuticals for Human Use (ICH) was borne as a response to these imperatives, and came into being in April 1990 in Brussels. This project was conceived with the notion of promoting a collaborative effort between the regulatory authorities of Europe, Japan and the United States in conjunction with experts from the pharmaceutical industry in these regions to discuss key scientific and technical elements related to product registration. The principles enumerated have become known as the GCP. It is hoped that harmonization will promote cost-effectiveness, minimize delay in the global development and availability of new medications and promote safeguards in drug deployment. Modern clinical trials frequently cite, as a part of the study protocol, that the trial will adhere to GCP norms.

Ethics in Medical Writing

Another area where ethical practices are essential, on the one hand, and controverted on the other is medical writing. Any written matter should be truthful, scientifically accurate and written in a way unintended to deceive or misinform. Examples of medical writing are not only medical journal articles or textbooks that all medical professionals are familiar with, but also medical articles in the lay press and advertising for medical products and services. In the West, there are established guidelines and regulations, sometimes backed by law, that protect the rights of the public and ensure that opportunities for misrepresentation are kept to the minimum. Elsewhere, particularly in the developing world, standards of self-policing tend to be lax and the quality of written matter is highly variable.

Medical journals maintain their standards through sound editorial policies, independence as far as possible from vested interests and the process of peer-review. As discussed in the chapter on research methodology, bias is a threat to the validity of a study. The process of peer-review at a journal typically entails the following steps:

1.   Submitted manuscript is reviewed by editorial staff. If deemed to be reasonably well prepared and of potential interest to the readers of the journal, the manuscript is sent out for "peer-review", typically with the names of the manuscript authors concealed. Peer-reviewers are generally practitioners with expertise in the fields dealt with by the journal, but are not directly affiliated with the journal, nor are they paid for their work. Peer-reviewers are not necessarily experts in research, but depending on the nature of the paper, the selected reviewers may have expertise and training in research methodology.

2.   Reviewers send back comments to the journal. They would make overall and specific comments, followed by a recommendation to publish, consider for publication with revisions or rejection. It would be quite unusual for an article to be recommended for publication without at least some minor revisions being requested.

3.   The journal editors contact the manuscript authors with these comments and the overall decision of the journal that would be one of the three possibilities outlined above. If the recommendation is for reconsideration with revisions, the editors ask the manuscript authors to resubmit, if they wish, within a specified time frame. Since this is usually an encouraging sign, most authors will go ahead and do so.

4. The journal reconsiders the revised manuscript and usually sends it back to the reviewers to see if they feel the revisions are acceptable. The reviewers send back their final comments and the journal takes a publication decision which is then communicated to the authors.

It can be readily seen that this painstaking and rigorous process tends to weed out poor articles and support the generation of higher quality work.

COPE Guidelines

In 1997, editors of a variety of prominent peer-reviewed medical journals based in UK and Europe came together in an important initiative to form the Committee On Publication Ethics (COPE) to provide a neutral venue and an explicit method for reviewing possible violations in ethical conduct of research and in publication. COPE put out guidelines that, as summarized on their website, address the following aspects: Study design and ethical approval, data analysis, authorship, conflict of interests, the peer review process, redundant publication, plagiarism, duties of editors, media relations, advertising, and how to deal with misconduct.

COPE also has formal meetings to adjudicate on cases of possible ethical misconduct referred to it for review. The full set of COPE guidelines are reproduced, with permission, at the end of the chapter (see Appendix 2.1).

The Medical Industry and Healthcare Providers– Where Is the Ethical Meeting Ground?

Much has been written about the relationship between industry and healthcare providers – in particular, relationship between physicians and the pharmaceutical industry. Research has clearly shown that despite protestations to the contrary from both sides, there are without doubt prescribing practices that favor existing relationships that a physician may have with a pharma company. It can seem perfectly logical from a business standpoint that a company selling a product (in this case, pharmaceuticals) would want to spend resources in trying to exert a positive influence on the decision-makers (in this case, the physician) to choose their products. The problem, however, is that this is one of the rare instances where the decision-maker is not the purchaser of the product – rather, it is actually the patient (or perhaps an insurer). Biased decisions taken by physicians in this context have repercussions not on themselves, but their patients. Thus, for example, if a physician prescribes an expensive antibiotic put out by a company whose rep just provided a nice lunch for his office staff, the patient ultimately picks up the tab. In this case, even though the doctor has not somehow siphoned money from the patient, nor has something necessarily illegal been done from the standpoint of medical ethics, this sort of deal-making is very troubling. Pharmaceutical funding of physicians CME is pervasive to the extent that both the content of CME programs and the nature of the attendees are heavily influenced by this largesse. There are a multitude of stories that have made the headlines (and many more that have not) of pharmaceutical companies giving extraordinary hospitality and benefits to physicians such as trips to swanky resorts (along with spouse) in the West, and in countries like India it is commonplace to hear of companies buying physicians groceries (and if need be refrigerators in which to store them), computers and even cars as signs of "appreciation"! Amidst growing international concern at this unholy nexus, and rumblings of legislation to stem the rot, pharmaceutical companies have moved to "regulate" themselves. On the face of it, this would seem a laudable thing but it seems undeniable that there is a degree of self-serving pragmatism in these maneuvers – seeking the high ground in the public relations battlefield and at the same time putting forth less onerous restrictions to stave off more painful ones imposed on these companies by the strong arm of the law. Some pharmaceutical sectors have national codes and complaint mechanisms such as those in Britain and Australia. For countries that have not developed national codes, two sets of international guidelines generally apply: (i) the World Health Organization's Criteria for Medicinal Drug Promotion and (ii) the Code of Pharmaceutical Marketing Practice put out by the International Federation of Pharmaceutical Manufacturers Associations. France has gone a step further by having a legal code that prohibits physicians from receiving gifts over a modest value or illegal payments. Violators are liable to face stiff fines or imprisonment up to two years.

While pharma guidelines tend to concentrate on rules to regulate their relationship with physicians, physicians' organizations in various countries also offer guidance about the proper conduct of commercially funded research. For instance, the Association of American Medical Colleges (AAMC) has issued two documents entitled Protecting subjects, preserving trust and promoting progress, one geared to academic institutions and the other to physicians. In 1990, the American College of Physicians put out guidelines which contain the yardstick (frequently quoted thereafter) for appropriateness as "Would you be willing to have these arrangements generally known?" A negative answer naturally implies the possibility of an ethically suspicious circumstance.

Warning Signs of an Unethical Milieu

Budding researchers, inexperienced in the ways of unethical practice, would be well advised to be alert to warning signals of a potentially unethical work environment to protect themselves from getting involved in unsavory situations that they may later come to regret:

- Funding from vested interests
- Pressure from vested interests to alter or dictate research related procedures
- Short-circuiting accepted procedures for human research, like submission of protocol to the institutional ethics committee
- Misrepresentation or falsification of data or material facts connected to the research
- Ultimately, the onus for fealty to the cardinal tenets of medical ethics falls on the physician/researcher – not on anyone else.

Ethics in Clinical Practice

Since the focus of this book is on research methodology and the techniques of evidence-based medicine, the important subject of clinical ethics will not be detailed here. There are excellent online resources that are available for free, some of which are listed under recommended resources. Practice in India is guided by the Indian Medical Council (Professional Conduct, Etiquette and Ethics) Regulations, 2002. Those found to be engaging in unethical practice are liable to have various forms of disciplinary action initiated against them, including but not limited to having their names removed from the medical register either for a specified period or permanently.

Acknowledgement

The author is grateful to the Committee On Publication Ethics (COPE) for permission to reproduce their guidelines.

Recommended Resources

Useful websites

1. Association of the British Pharmaceutical Industry: www.abpi.org.uk
2. American Academy of Pharmaceutical Physicians: www.aapp.org
3. American College of Physicians: www.acponline.org
4. American Medical Association: www.ama-assn.org
5. Association of American Medical Colleges: www.aamc.org
6. Australian Medical Association: www.ama.com.au
7. British Association of Pharmaceutical Physicians: www.brapp.org.uk
8. Conseil National de l'Ordre des Médecins: www.conseil-national.medecin.fr
9. Committee on Publication Ethics: www.publicationethics.org.uk
10. Good Publication Practice for Pharmaceutical Companies: www.gpp-guidelines.org
11. Indian Council of Medical Research: http://icmr.nic.in/
12. International Committee of Medical Journal Editors: www.icmje.org
13. International Conference on Harmonisation of Technical Requirements for Registration of Pharmaceuticals for Human Use: www.ich.org
14. International Federation of Pharmaceutical Manufacturers Associations: www.ifpma.org
15. International Federation of Associations of Pharmaceutical Physicians: www.ifapp.org
16. Medical Council of India: www.mciindia.org
17. Medicines Australia: www.medicinesaustralia.com.au
18. No free lunch: www.nofreelunch.org
19. Pharmaceutical Research and Manufacturers of America: www.phrma.org
20. World Health Organization: www.who.int
21. World Medical Association: www.wma.net

Articles

1. Abbasi K, Smith R. No more free lunches. *BMJ.* 2003;326: 1155-6.
2. Lexchin J, Light DW. Commercial influence and the content of medical journals. *BMJ.* 2006;332: 1444-46.
3. Wager E. How to dance with porcupines: rules and guidelines on doctors' relations with drug companies. *BMJ.* 2003;326: 1196-8.

4. Lewis S, Baird P, Evans RG, Ghali WA, Wright CJ, Gibson E, et al. Dancing with the porcupine: rules for governing the university-industry relationship. *CMAJ*. 2001;165:783.

5. Simmonds H. Complaints about advertising of medicines are encouraged. *BMJ*. 2002;324: 850-1.

6. American College of Physicians. Physicians and the pharmaceutical industry. *Ann Intern Med*. 1990;112: 624-6.

7. Coyle SL. Physician-industry relations: part 1: individual physicians. *Ann Intern Med*. 2002;136: 396-402.

8. Coyle SL. Physician-industry relations: part 2: organizational issues. *Ann Intern Med*. 2002;136: 403-6.

9. Davidoff F, DeAngelis CD, Drazen JM, Hoey J, Højgaard L, Horton R, et al. Sponsorship, authorship, and accountability. *Ann Intern Med*. 2001;135: 463-6.

10. Smith R. Maintaining the integrity of the scientific record. *BMJ*. 2001;323: 588.

APPENDIX 2.1

Committee on Publication Ethics (COPE): Guidelines on Good Publication Practice

Why the Guidelines were Developed

Cope was founded in 1997 to address breaches of research and publication ethics. A voluntary body providing a discussion forum and advice for scientific editors, it aims to find practical ways of dealing with the issues, and to develop good practice.

We thought it essential to attempt to define best practice in the ethics of scientific publishing. These guidelines should be useful for authors, editors, editorial board members, readers, owners of journals, and publishers.

Intellectual honesty should be actively encouraged in all medical and scientific courses of study, and used to inform publication ethics and prevent misconduct. It is with that in mind that these guidelines have been produced.

Details of other guidelines on the ethics of research and published codes of conduct are listed in the Appendix.

How the Guidelines were Developed

The guidelines were developed from a preliminary version drafted by individual members of the committee, which was then submitted to extensive consultation. They address: study design and ethical approval, data analysis, authorship, conflict of interests, the peer review process, redundant publication, plagiarism, duties of editors, media relations, advertising, and how to deal with misconduct.

What they aim to do

These guidelines are intended to be advisory rather than prescriptive, and to evolve over time. We hope that they will be disseminated widely, endorsed by editors, and refined by those who use them.

I. Study Design and Ethical Approval

Definition

Good research should be well justified, well planned, appropriately designed, and ethically approved. To conduct research to a lower standard may constitute misconduct.

Action

1. Laboratory and clinical research should be driven by protocol; pilot studies should have a written rationale.
2. Research protocols should seek to answer specific questions, rather than just collect data.
3. Protocols must be carefully agreed by all contributors and collaborators, including, if appropriate, the participants.
4. The final protocol should form part of the research record.
5. Early agreement on the precise roles of the contributors and collaborators, and on matters of authorship and publication, is advised.
6. Statistical issues should be considered early in study design, including power calculations, to ensure there are neither too few nor too many participants.
7. Formal and documented ethical approval from an appropriately constituted research ethics committee is required for all studies involving people, medical records, and anonymised human tissues.
8. Use of human tissues in research should conform to the highest ethical standards, such as those recommended by the Nuffield Council on Bioethics.
9. Fully informed consent should always be sought. It may not always be possible, however, and in such circumstances, an appropriately constituted research ethics committee should decide if this is ethically acceptable.
10. When participants are unable to give fully informed consent, research should follow international guidelines, such as those of the Council for International Organizations of Medical Sciences (CIOMS).
11. Animal experiments require full compliance with local, national, ethical, and regulatory principles, and local licensing arrangements. International standards vary.
12. Formal supervision, usually the responsibility of the principal investigator, should be provided for all research projects: this must include quality control, and the frequent review and long term retention (may be up to 15 years) of all records and primary outputs.

II. Data Analysis

Definition

Data should be appropriately analyzed, but inappropriate analysis does not necessarily amount to misconduct. Fabrication and falsification of data do constitute misconduct.

Action

1. All sources and methods used to obtain and analyze data, including any electronic pre-processing, should be fully disclosed; detailed explanations should be provided for any exclusions.
2. Methods of analysis must be explained in detail, and referenced, if they are not in common use.
3. The post hoc analysis of subgroups is acceptable, as long as this is disclosed. Failure to disclose that the analysis was post hoc is unacceptable.
4. The discussion section of a paper should mention any issues of bias, which have been considered, and explain how they have been dealt with in the design and interpretation of the study.

III. Authorship

Definition

There is no universally agreed definition of authorship, although attempts have been made (see Appendix). As a minimum, authors should take responsibility for a particular section of the study.

Action

1. The award of authorship should balance intellectual contributions to the conception, design, analysis and writing of the study against the collection of data and other routine work. If there is no task that can reasonably be attributed to a particular individual, then that individual should not be credited with authorship.
2. To avoid disputes over attribution of academic credit, it is helpful to decide early on in the planning of a research project who will be credited as authors, as contributors, and who will be acknowledged.
3. All authors must take public responsibility for the content of their paper. The multidisciplinary nature of much research can make

this difficult, but this can be resolved by the disclosure of individual contributions.

4. Careful reading of the target journal's "Advice to Authors" is advised, in the light of current uncertainties.

IV. Conflicts of Interest

Definition

Conflicts of interest comprise those which may not be fully apparent and which may influence the judgement of author, reviewers, and editors.

They have been described as those which, when revealed later, would make a reasonable reader feel misled or deceived. They may be personal, commercial, political, academic or financial.

'Financial' interests may include employment, research funding, stock or share ownership, payment for lectures or travel, consultancies and company support for staff.

Action

1. Such interests, where relevant, must be declared to editors by researchers, authors, and reviewers.
2. Editors should also disclose relevant conflicts of interest to their readers. If in doubt, disclose. Sometimes editors may need to withdraw from the review and selection process for the relevant submission.

V. Peer Review

Definition

Peer reviewers are external experts chosen by editors to provide written opinions, with the aim of improving the study.

Working methods vary from journal to journal, but some use open procedures in which the name of the reviewer is disclosed, together with the full or 'edited' report.

Action

1. Suggestions from authors as to who might act as reviewers are often useful, but there should be no obligations on editors to use those suggested.
2. The duty of confidentiality in the assessment of a manuscript must be maintained by expert reviewers, and this extends to

reviewers' colleagues who may be asked (with the editor's permission) to give opinions on specific sections.

3. The submitted manuscript should not be retained or copied.
4. Reviewers and editors should not make any use of the data, arguments, or interpretations, unless they have the authors' permission.
5. Reviewers should provide speedy, accurate, courteous, unbiased and justifiable reports.
6. If reviewers suspect misconduct, they should write in confidence to the editor.
7. Journals should publish accurate descriptions of their peer review, selection, and appeals processes.
8. Journals should also provide regular audits of their acceptance rates and publication times.

VI. Redundant Publication

Definition

Redundant publication occurs when two or more papers, without full cross reference, share the same hypothesis, data, discussion points, or conclusions.

Action

1. Published studies do not need to be repeated unless further confirmation is required.
2. Previous publication of an abstract during the proceedings of meetings does not preclude subsequent submission for publication, but full disclosure should be made at the time of submission.
3. Re-publication of a paper in another language is acceptable, provided that there is full and prominent disclosure of its original source at the time of submission.
4. At the time of submission, authors should disclose details of related papers, even if in a different language, and similar papers in press.

VII. Plagiarism

Definition

Plagiarism ranges from the unreferenced use of others' published and unpublished ideas, including research grant applications to submission under "new" authorship of a complete paper, sometimes in a different language.

It may occur at any stage of planning, research, writing, or publication; it applies to print and electronic versions.

Action

1. All sources should be disclosed, and if large amounts of other people's written or illustrative material are to be used, permission must be sought.

VIII. Duties of Editors

Definition

Editors are the stewards of journals. They usually take over their journal from the previous editor(s) and always want to hand over the journal in good shape.

Most editors provide direction for the journal and build a strong management team.

They must consider and balance the interests of many constituents, including readers, authors, staff, owners, editorial board members, advertisers and the media.

Action

1. Editors' decisions to accept or reject a paper for publication should be based only on the paper's importance, originality, and clarity, and the study's relevance to the remit of the journal.
2. Studies that challenge previous work published in the journal should be given an especially sympathetic hearing.
3. Studies reporting negative results should not be excluded.
4. All original studies should be peer reviewed before publication, taking into full·account possible bias due to related or conflicting interests.
5. Editors must treat all submitted papers as confidential.
6. When a published paper is subsequently found to contain major flaws, editors must accept responsibility for correcting the record prominently and promptly.

IX. Media Relations

Definition

Medical research findings are of increasing interest to the print and broadcast media.

Journalists may attend scientific meetings, at which preliminary research findings are presented, leading to their premature publication in the mass media.

Action

1. Authors approached by the media should give as balanced an account of their work as possible, ensuring that they point out where evidence ends and speculations begins.
2. Simultaneous publication in the mass media and a peer reviewed journal is advised, as this usually means that enough evidence and data have been provided to satisfy informed and critical readers.
3. Where this is not possible, authors should help journalists to produce accurate reports, but refrain from supplying additional data.
4. All efforts should be made to ensure that patients who have helped with the research should be informed of the results by the authors before the mass media, especially if there are clinical implications.
5. Authors should be advised by the organizers if journalists are to attend scientific meetings.
6. It may be helpful to authors to be advised of any media policies operated by the journal in which their work is to be published.

X. Advertising

Definition

Many scientific journals and meetings derive significant income form advertising. Reprints may also be lucrative.

Action

1. Editorial decisions must not be influenced by advertising revenue or reprint potential: editorial and advertising administration must be clearly separated.

2. Advertisements that mislead must be refused, and editors must be willing to publish criticisms, according to the same criteria used for material in the rest of the journal.
3. Reprints should be published as they appear in the journal unless a correction is to be added.

Dealing with Misconduct

1. Principles

1. The general principle confirming misconduct is intention to cause others to regard as true that which is not true.
2. The examination of misconduct must therefore focus, not only on the particular act or omission, but also on the intention of the researcher, author, editor, reviewer or publisher involved.
3. Deception may be by intention, by reckless disregard of possible consequences, or by negligence. It is implicit, therefore, that 'best practice' requires complete honesty, with full disclosure.
4. Codes of practice may raise awareness, but can never be exhaustive.

2. Investigating misconduct

1. Editors should not simply reject papers that raise questions of misconduct. They are ethically obliged to pursue the case. However, knowing how to investigate and respond to possible cases of misconduct is difficult.
2. COPE is always willing to advice, but for legal reasons, can only advise on anonymised cases.
3. It is for the editor to decide what action to take.

3. Serious misconduct

1. Editors must take all allegations and suspicions of misconduct seriously, but they must recognize that they do not usually have either the legal legitimacy or the means to conducts investigations to serious cases.
2. The editor must decide when to alert the employers of the accused author(s).
3. Some evidence is required, but if employers have a process for investigating accusations - as they are increasingly required to do—then editors do not need to assemble a complete case.

Indeed, it may be ethically unsound for editors to do so, because such action usually means consulting experts, so spreading abroad serious questions about the author(s).

4. If editors are presented with convincing evidence perhaps by reviewers – of serious misconduct, they should immediately pass this on to the employers, notifying the author(s) that they are doing so.

5. If accusations of serious misconduct are not accompanied by convincing evidence, then editors should confidentially seek expert advice.

6. If the experts raise serious questions about the research, then editors should notify the employers.

7. If the experts find no evidence of misconduct, the editorial processes should proceed in the normal way.

8. If presented with convincing evidence of serious misconduct, where there is no employer to whom this can be referred, and the author(s) are registered doctors, cases can be referred to the General Medical Council.

9. If, however, there is no organization with the legitimacy and the means to conduct an investigation, then the editor may decide that the case is sufficiently important to warrant publishing something in the journal. Legal advice will then be essential.

10. If editors are convinced that an employer has not conducted an adequate investigation of a serious accusation, they may feel that publication of a notice in the journal is warranted. Legal advice will be essential.

11. Authors should be given the opportunity to respond to accusations of serious misconduct.

4. Less serious misconduct

1. Editors may judge that it is not necessary to involve employers in less serious cases of misconduct, such as redundant publication, deception over authorship, or failure to declare conflict of interest. Sometimes the evidence may speak for itself, although it may be wise to appoint an independent expert.

2. Editors should remember that accusations of even minor misconduct may have serious implications for the author(s), and it may then be necessary to ask the employers to investigate.

3. Authors should be given the opportunity to respond to any charge of minor misconduct.

4. If convinced of wrongdoing, editors may wish to adopt some of the sanctions outlined below.

5. Sanctions

1. Sanctions may be applied separately or combined. The following are ranked in approximate order of severity:
2. A letter of explanation (and education) to the authors, where there appears to be a genuine misunderstanding of principles.
3. A letter of reprimand and warning as to future conduct.
4. A formal letter to the relevant head of institution or funding body.
5. Publication of a notice of redundant publication or plagiarism.
6. An editorial giving full details of the misconduct.
7. Refusal to accept future submissions from the individual, unit, or institution responsible for the misconduct, for a stated period.
8. Formal withdrawal or retraction of the paper from the scientific literature, informing other editors and the indexing authorities.
9. Reporting the case to the General Medical Council, or other such authority or organization which can investigate and act with due process.

Appendix

- The Association of the British Pharmaceutical Industry. *Facilities for nonpatient volunteer studies.* London: PBI, 1989.
- The Association of the British Pharmaceutical Industry. *Guidelines for medical experiments in nonpatient human volunteers.* London: ABPI, 1990.
- ABPI fact sheets and guidance notes: *Clinical trials and compensation guidelines,* January 1991. *Guidelines for phase IV clinical trials,* September 1993. *Guidelines on the conduct of investigator site audits,* January 1994. *Relationship between the medical profession and the pharmaceutical industry,* June 1994. *Good clinical trial practice,* November 1995. *Patient information and consents for clinical trials,* May 1997. *Guidelines on the structure of a formal agreement to conduct sponsored clinical research,* July 1998. *Good clinical research practice,* July 1998.
- Council for International Organizations of Medical Sciences (CIOMS). *International Guidelines for Ethical review of Epidemiological Studies.* Geneva: WHO, 1991.
- General Medical Council. Good medical practice guidelines series: *Consent,* February 1999. *Confidentiality,* October 1995. *Transplantation of organs from live donors,* November 1992.

- International Committee of Medical journal Editors (ICMJE). Uniform requirements for manuscripts submitted to biomedical journals. JAMA, 277: 927-934, 1997.
- Medical Research Council. *Policy and procedure for inquiring into allegations of scientific misconduct.* London: MRC, 1997.
- Medical Research Council. *The ethical conduct of research on the mentally incapacitated.* London: MCR, 1991.
- Medical Research Council. *The ethical conduct of research on children.* London: MRC, 1991.
- Medical Research Council. *Responsibility in the use of animals in medical research.* London: MCR, 1993.
- Medical Research Council. *Responsibility in the use of personal medical information for research. Principles and guidelines to practice.* London: MCR, 1985.
- Medical Research Council. *MCR Guidelines for good clinical practice in clinical trials.* London: MCR, 1998.
- Medical Research Council. *Principles in the assessment and conduct of medical research and publicising results.* London: MCR, 1995.
- Nuffield Council on Bioethics. *Human tissue: Ethical and legal issues.* London: Nuffield Council on Bioethics, 1995.
- Royal College of Physicians. *Research involving patients.* London: RCP, 1990.

Acknowledgement

The following are gratefully acknowledged for their contribution to the drafting of these guidelines:
- Philip Fulford (Coordinator)
- Professor Michael Doherty
- Ms Jane Smith
- Dr Richard Smith
- Dr Fiona Godlee
- Dr Peter Wilmshurst
- Dr Richard Horton
- Professor Michael Farthing
- Other members of COPE
- Delegates to the Meeting on April 27 1999
- Other corresponding editors

3

Introduction to Biostatistics

R. Vinaitheerthan and Ajit N. Babu

- *Need for Biostatistical Tools*
- *Use of Biostatistical Tools in Planning Research*
- *Classification of Variables*
- *Statistical Hypothesis*
- *Data Collection and Analysis*
- *Descriptive Data Analysis*
- *Relationships between Two Variables*
- *Statistical Distributions*
- *Inferential Data Analysis*
- *Survival Analysis*

Statistics can be defined as the science of collecting, organizing, analyzing and interpreting data; when applied to biological problems, it is known as *biostatistics*. The role of biostatistics is vital in every stage of research, from conception of research idea to the final analysis of results obtained. Therefore, a basic knowledge of biostatistics is essential to be a successful researcher. This chapter examines basic biostatistical principles and explores their application with relevant examples.

Need for Biostatistical Tools

Biostatistical tools are necessary in research, since it is almost impossible to study an entire population because of the scarcity of resources, such as money, time, etc., or due to a desire to expose only the minimal number of subjects to the risks involved in certain clinical trials. When an entire population cannot be studied, then a part of the population (i.e. a sample) is examined.

When the researcher studies the sample and draws inferences about the population, serious errors can result if the sample is not truly representative of the larger population. Biostatistical tools help the researcher to overcome this bias and help draw valid conclusions about the population with a defined level of confidence. Biostatistics has a role in each phase of the research. Let us start with the first stage of research — planning.

Use of Biostatistical Tools in Planning Research

After identifying and defining the problem, the researcher decides on the type of study design to follow. Once the type of study design is finalized, the variables have to be identified and classified before proceeding to the next step of developing a hypothesis in the case of an experimental study. The variables can be categorized by their nature, type and scales of measurement, i.e., independent or dependent, quantitative or qualitative, scales of measurement such as nominal, ordinal, interval and ratio scales, and so on. The nature of the variables will have a significant effect on data collection and analysis.

Classification of Variables

Classification of Variables According to their Nature

Independent variables

Variables that can either be manipulated by the researcher or variables that are not outcomes of the study but still affect its results are called *independent variables*. A good example is age of the subjects, which can be an independent variable that may affect a study outcome variable, such as subject survival.

Dependent variables

The outcome variables defined as part of the research process are termed *dependent variables* and these will be affected by the independent variables under study. An example of a dependant variable can be the number of people who developed a particular disease in a cohort study.

Classification of Variables According to their Type

Quantitative variables

Variables that can be measured numerically are called *quantitative variables*. These variables can be further classified as *continuous* and *discrete* variables. A continuous variable could take any value in an interval. Examples of continuous data are findings for measurements like body mass, height, blood pressure or serum cholesterol. Discrete variables will have whole integer values. Their examples are the number of hospitalizations per patient in a year or the number of hypoglycemic events recorded in a diabetic patient over 6 months.

Qualitative variables

Variables that cannot be measured numerically are called qualitative variables. An example is gender.

Classification of Variables According to the Scale of Measurement

Nominal scale variables

Nominal scale measurements can only be classified but not put into an order, and mathematical functions cannot be performed on them. Gender is an example for this sort of variable as well.

Ordinal scale variables

These variables can be put into a definite order, but the difference between two positions in the ordinal scale does not have a quantitative meaning. Essentially, this scale is a form of ranking. An example is the military hierarchy, where a general outranks a colonel, who in turn outranks a captain. Though there is a clear series of ranks, the relationship is not numerical.

Interval scale variables

In an interval measurement scale, one unit on the scale represents the same magnitude of the characteristic being measured across the whole range of the scale, i.e., the intervals between the numbers are equal. However, the *ratio* between set of two numbers in the scale is not equal, because an interval scale lacks a true zero point.

Temperature in Fahrenheit would be a perfect example for interval scale, because though we can add and subtract degrees (70° is 10° warmer than 60°), we cannot multiply values or create ratios (70° is not twice as warm as 35°).

Ratio scale variables

Ratio scale variables will have all the properties of interval variables with the ratio between two numbers in the ratio scales being identical. Ratio scales have an absolute or zero point. For example, a 100-year old person is indeed twice as old as a 50-year old one

Statistical Hypothesis

After identifying and defining the variables to be investigated, the researcher has to develop the study hypothesis, if an experimental study is to be conducted. Classically, such studies will have two hypotheses. One is a *null hypothesis*, which is a statement of no effect or no association, while the *alternative hypothesis* is a statement that depicts the researcher's interest or scientific belief.

To illustrate, let us take the case when a researcher wants to test whether a form of chemotherapy for treating small cell lung cancer is more effective than the standard therapy. The researcher can formulate the null and alternative hypothesis as follows:

Null hypothesis: There is no difference in efficacy between the standard therapy and the new therapy.

Alternative hypothesis: New therapy is superior to the standard therapy.

Two types of errors can occur while making conclusions regarding the null hypothesis: **Type I error** and **Type II error**. A Type I error refers to rejecting the null hypothesis when the null hypothesis is true (false positive). A Type II error refers to accepting the null hypothesis when it is actually false (false negative).

Level of Significance and Power of the Test

The probability of making a Type I error is called level of significance (α). Normally, researchers would aim to minimize the probability of making a Type I error. Most researchers will set this probability to 0.05.

The probability of making a Type II error is (β). The power of the study is calculated from (1-β) and is defined as the probability of detecting a real difference when the null hypothesis is false.

These parameters have to be predetermined by the researcher, prior to the study to avert the risk of erroneously accepting the null hypothesis (even though it is really false) due to an inadequate sample size that is not enough to detect a true difference.

Once the hypothesis, level of significance and power of the study have been fixed, the researcher can proceed to determine the statistical processes for the proper conduct and analysis of the study.

Determining the Sample Size for the Study

As discussed earlier, the researcher usually draws conclusions about the population from a small part of it – the sample. The information collected from the sample is known as sample statistics, which is used to estimate the characteristics of the unknown population, i.e., population parameters.

We know that the sample taken from the population should accurately represent the population under study. To get a representative sample, the most important intervention is to select a sample large enough to adequately represent the population. Sadly, researchers have to strike a balance between striving for maximal validity and keeping the cost of the study at a level they can afford...!

From what has been stated so far, it can be deduced that the sampling process involves two important aspects. One is deciding the method of sampling and the other is determining the sample size for the study.

Method of sampling

Method of sampling involves selection of samples from the given population. There are two basic methods in sampling: (a) probability sampling and (b) non-probability sampling.

a. **Probability sampling:**
   • Simple random sampling
   • Stratified random sampling
   • Systematic sampling
   • Cluster sampling

b. **Non-probability sampling:**
   • Judgement sampling
   • Convenience sampling

Sample size

Determination of the sample size is based on a number of issues such as:

- Type of study
- Nature of study, i.e., whether estimating parameters or comparing parameters
- Type of sampling method
- Type of analysis used in the study
- Power of the study
- Effect size
- Study budget
- Time factor

It can be readily appreciated that sample size calculation is rather complex. It is always best to consult a statistician for determination of sample size and other challenging biostatistical issues when embarking on a research project.

Data Collection and Analysis

Data Collection

After determining the sample size the researcher then proceeds to collect data. Data can be gathered through primary or secondary sources.

Primary sources

Primary sources are original materials collected by the investigator himself. While collecting the primary data, the researcher can use the following methods.

- Personal interview
- Telephone interview
- Face to face administration of questionnaire
- Mailing questionnaire by post
- Mailing questionnaire by email
- Online data collection through websites
- Data collected through experimentation
- Data collected through observation by the researcher

Each of the above methods has its advantages and limitations. A rule of thumb is to verify 5% of the data as a quality control measure to validate the data.

Secondary sources

Secondary data is that which has been collected by individuals or agencies for purposes other than those of our particular research study. For example, if a government department has conducted a survey of, say, family health expenditures, then a health insurance company might use this data in the organization's evaluations of the total potential market for a new insurance product.

Examples of secondary sources are:

- Bibliographies
- Online databases
- Biographies
- Textbooks
- Handbooks and manuals
- Review articles and editorials

Data Compilation

Once the data are collected and validated, these can then be compiled. Tabulation is the basic method of compilation.

Data Analysis

Primary data analysis starts with the diagrammatic and graphical representation of the data. The following are frequently used methods for data analysis:

A. Histogram
B. Bar graph
C. Pie chart
D. Line graph

A. Histogram

Histograms consist of a series of blocks or bars, each with an area proportional to the frequency of occurrence of a particular value. In a

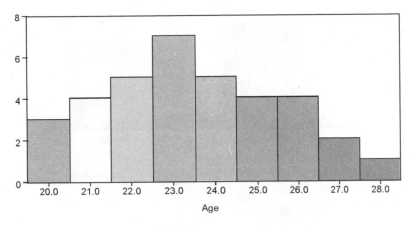

Fig. 3.1. Age distribution of patients in a cancer study

histogram the horizontal scale is used for the variable and the vertical scale to show the frequency (Fig. 3.1).

The highest block in a histogram indicates the most frequent values. The lowest blocks show the least frequent values. Where there are no blocks, there are no results corresponding to those values. Blocks of equal height indicate that the values they represent occur in the same frequency.

B. Bar graph

In a simple bar chart, each bar represents a different group of data. Although the bars may be drawn either vertically or horizontally, it is conventional to draw the bars vertically whenever possible. The height or length of the bar is drawn in proportion to the size of the group of data being represented. Unlike a histogram, the bars are separated from one another (Fig.3.2).

C. Pie charts

Pie charts, or circle graphs as they are sometimes known, are very different from other types of graphs. They do not use a set of axes to plot points. Pie charts display percentages.

The circle of a pie graph represents 100%. Each portion that takes up space within the circle stands for a part of that 100%. In this way, it is possible to see how something is divided among different groups (Fig. 3.3).

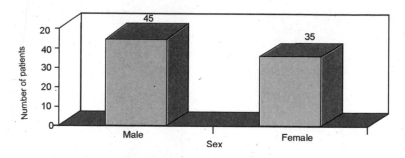

Fig. 3.2. Gender distribution of patients in a cancer study

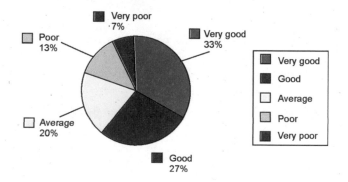

Fig. 3.3. Patient satisfaction with care

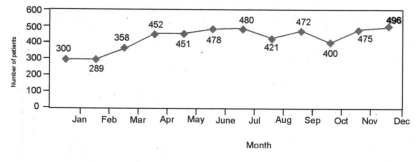

Fig. 3.4. Outpatients visited during the year 2006

D. Line graph

A Line graph is drawn after plotting points corresponding to different values on a graph that are then connected by a line. Line graphs are useful in displaying data trends (Fig. 3.4).

Descriptive Data Analysis

The next stage of data analysis consists of descriptive and inferential data analysis. Descriptive data analysis provides the researcher a basic picture of the problem he is studying. It consists of:

Measures of Central Tendency

A measure of central tendency is a value that represents a typical or central element of a data set. The important measures of central tendency are: (a) mean, (b) median and (c) mode.

a. Mean

Mean (average) is the sum of the data entries divided by the number of entries. The sample mean is denoted by $\overline{X}$ and the population mean is denoted by μ.

Population mean
$$\mu = \Sigma\, x/N$$
Where N is the number of items in the population

Sample mean
$$\overline{X} = \Sigma\, x/n$$
Where n is the number of items in the sample

Properties of mean

- Data possessing an interval scale or a ratio scale, usually have a mean.
- All the values are included in computing the mean.
- A given set of data has a unique mean.
- The mean is affected by unusually large or small data values (known as outliers).
- The arithmetic mean is the only measure of central tendency where the sum of the deviations of different values from the mean in the given dataset is zero.

b. Median

The median of a data set is the middle data entry when the data set is sorted in order. If the data set contains an even number of elements, the median is the mean of the two middle entries. The median is the most appropriate measure of central tendency to use when the data under consideration are ranked data, rather than quantitative data.

c. Mode

The mode of a data set is the entry that occurs with the greatest frequency. A set may have no mode or may be bimodal when two entries each occur with the same greatest frequency. The mode is most useful when an important aspect of describing the data involves determining the number of times each value occurs. If the data are qualitative, then mode is particularly useful. Table 3.1 gives an overview of the measures of central tendency appropriate for different data measurement scales.

Table 3.1: Measures of central tendency for different measurement scales

	Nominal	Ordinal	Interval	Ratio
Mean			X	X
Median		X		
Mode	X			

Measures of Dispersion

Measures of dispersion indicate the amount of variation or spread in a data set. There are four important measures of dispersion:

a. Range
b. Interquartile range
c. Variance
d. Standard deviation

a. The range

- The *range* is the difference between the largest and the smallest observation.
- The range is very sensitive to extreme values, because it uses only the extreme values on each end of the ordered array.
- The range completely ignores the distribution of data.

b. The interquartile range

- The *interquartile range* (midspread) is the difference between the third and first quartiles.
- Interquartile range $= Q_3 - Q_1$.
- The interquartile range gives the range of the middle 50% of the data.
- It is not affected by extreme values.
- It ignores the distribution of data within the sample.

c. Variance

The variance is the average of the squared differences between each observation and the mean.

d. Standard deviation

Standard deviation is the square root of the sample variance.

Properties of standard deviation

It lends itself to further mathematical analysis in a way that the range cannot, because the standard deviation can be used in calculating other statistics. It is worth noting that the standard deviation for nominal or ordinal data cannot be measured because it is not possible to calculate a mean for such data.

Measures of Skewness

Skewness is a measure of lack of symmetry of a distribution. There are two types of skewed distributons — one is negatively skewed (left skewness) and the other is positively skewed (right skewed) (Fig. 3.5).

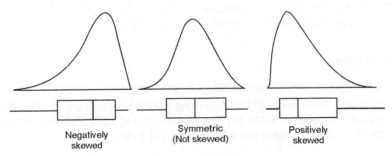

Negatively skewed   Symmetric (Not skewed)   Positively skewed

Fig. 3.5. Skewed distributions of data

When the researcher encounters this kind of situation, he can use log transformation on the variable to make the distribution symmetrical.

- In a symmetrical distribution the mean, median, and mode will have the same value and skewness will be equal to 0.
- A positive skewness means the shape of the distribution will be skewed right and mode < median < mean.
- In a distribution with negative skewness, mean < median < mode.

Measures of Kurtosis

Kurtosis is a measure of "peakedness" of a distribution. There are three types of kurtosis: mesokurtic, leptokurtic and platykurtic (Fig. 3.6). The leptokurtic is known as positive kurtosis while platykurtic is termed negative kurtosis. When the distribution is normal, then the kurtosis is called mesokurtic.

Further details about skewness and kurtosis can be found in more specialized works on Biostatistics.

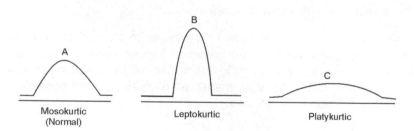

Fig. 3.6. Different types of kurtosis in data distribution

Relationships between Two Variables

Two of the important techniques used to study the relationship between two variables are correlation and regression.

Correlation

- It measures association between two variables.
- In graph form, it would be shown as a 'scatter diagram' putting the scores for one variable on the horizontal (X) axis and the values for the other variable on the vertical (Y) axis.

- The pattern shows the strength of the association between the two variables and also whether it is a 'positive' or a 'negative' relationship.
- A 'positive' relationship means that as the value of one variable increases so does the value of the other variable.
- A 'negative' relationship means that as the value of one variable increases, the value of the other variable decreases.

Measures of correlation

There are two measures of correlation. One is Pearson's product-moment correlation (r) and the other is Spearman's rank order co-efficient (rho). Both the measures will tell us only how closely the two variables are connected, but they cannot tell us whether one causes the other. Correlation values can range from −1 to +1.

Interpretation of correlation value

Correlation value	Interpretation
Equal to 0	no correlation
Less than 0.2	correlation is very low
Between 0.2 and 0.4	correlation is low
Between 0.41 and 0.70	correlation is moderate
Between 0.71 and 0.90	correlation is high
Over 0.91	correlation is very high
Equal to 1	perfect correlation

Scatter diagram

Scatter diagrams can also be used to depict the correlation between two variables. The greater the spread/scatter, the lower will be the correlation value. The following scatter diagram (Fig. 3.7) shows the correlation between age and weight in a cancer study.

By merely inspecting the diagram we can infer that there is low correlation between the two variables, because the spread is large while the location of the scatter plot towards the upper right tells us that whatever correlation may exist is likely to be positive. The Pearson correlation coefficient for the same data was determined to be 0.196, which confirms a very low positive correlation.

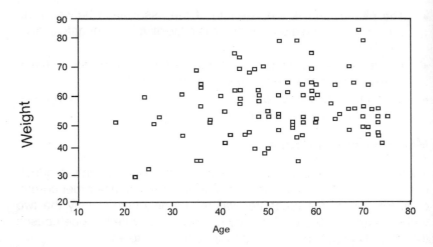

Fig. 3.7. Scatter diagram showing correlation between age and weight in a cancer study

Properties of correlation

- Correlation will not establish a cause and effect relationship.
- Correlation may sometimes be a non-sense correlation.
- It is very sensitive to extreme values.

Simple Regression Analysis

It gives the equation of a straight line and enables prediction of the value of one variable from that of the other. Normally, the dependent variable is plotted on the Y axis and the independent variable on the X axis. There are three major assumptions. First, any values of x and y are normally distributed. Second, the variability of y should be the same for each value of y. Third; the relationship between the two variables is linear.

The equation of a regression line is: "y=a + bx", where 'a' is the intercept, 'b' is the slope, 'x' is the independent variable and 'y' is the dependent variable. The slope 'b' is sometimes called regression coefficient and it has the same sign as correlation co-efficient (i.e., 'r').

Probability

- Probability is defined as the likelihood of an event or outcome in a trial.

$$p(A) \frac{\text{Number of outcomes classified as A}}{\text{Total Number of possible outcomes}}$$

Statistical Distributions

Statistical distributions are classified into two categories: discrete and continuous.

Discrete Distributions

Binomial distribution

It describes the possible number of times that a particular event will occur in a sequence of observations. The event is coded in a binary fashion, i.e., it may or may not occur. The binomial distribution is used when a researcher is interested in investigating the occurrence of an event, not its magnitude. For instance, in a clinical trial, a patient may survive or die. The researcher studies only the number of survivors, not how long the patient survives after treatment.

Poisson distribution

The Poisson distribution is an appropriate model for count data. Examples of such data are number of deaths due to vehicular accidents in a city, the number of printing errors in a textbook or the number of leucocytes seen in a peripheral smear under a microscope.

Continuous Distributions

Normal distribution

The normal distribution (also called a Gaussian distribution) is a symmetric, bell-shaped distribution with a single peak (Fig. 3.8). Its peak corresponds to the mean, median and mode of the distribution. Normal distribution is characterized by two numbers. Mean gives the location of the peak, and the standard deviation gives the width of the peak.

A data set that satisfies the following four criteria is likely to have a nearly normal distribution:

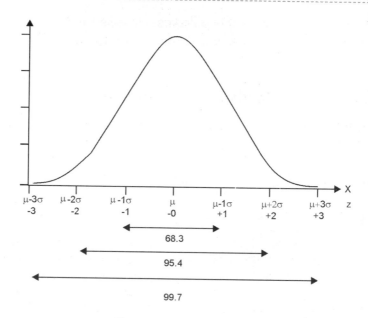

Fig. 3.8. Normal distribution

1. Data in a normal distribution are clustered around the mean resulting in a single peak.
2. Data in a normal distribution are evenly spread around the mean and this makes the distribution symmetric.
3. In such a distribution, only a small number of values will substantially deviate from the mean, thus giving thin tails.
4. Variation in individual data values may occur due to the influence of intrinsic or extrinsic factors.

The 68-95-99.7 Rules for a Normal Distribution:

- About 68.3% of the data in a normally distributed data set will fall within 1 standard deviation of the mean.
- About 95.4% of the data in a normally distributed data set will fall within 2 standard deviations of the mean.
- About 99.7% of the data in a normally distributed data set will fall within 3 standard deviations of the mean.

Inferential Data Analysis

As the researcher draws scientific conclusions from his study using only a sample instead of the whole population, he can justify his conclusion with help of statistical inference tools. The principal concepts involved in statistical inference are theory of estimation and hypothesis testing.

Theory of Estimation

- **Point estimation:** A single value is used to provide the best estimate of the parameter of interest.

- **Interval estimation:** Interval estimates shows the estimate of the parameter and also give an idea of the confidence that the researcher has in that estimate. This leads us to consideration of confidence intervals.

Confidence interval (CI)

A *confidence interval estimate* of a parameter consists of an interval, along with a probability that the interval contains the unknown parameter. The **level of confidence** in a confidence interval is a probability that represents the percentage of intervals that will contain the parameter if a large number of repeated samples are obtained. The level of confidence is denoted $(1-\alpha)$ 100%.

The narrower the width of the confidence interval, the lower is the error of the point estimate it contains. The sample size, sample variance and the level of confidence all affect the width of the confidence interval.

- If the sample size increases, it will decrease the width of the confidence interval.
- If the level of confidence increases, the width will increase.
- If the variation in sample increase, it will increases the width of confidence interval

Confidence intervals can be computed for estimating single mean and proportions and also for comparing the difference between two means or proportions. Confidence interval (CI) is widely used to represent the main clinical outcomes instead of p values, as CI has many advantages over p values (such as giving information about effect size, variability and possible range). The most commonly used confidence interval is the 95% CI. Increasingly, medical journals and publications require authors to calculate and report the 95% CI wherever appropriate, since it gives a measure of the range of effect sizes possible – information that is of great relevance to clinicians. The term 95% CI means that it is the interval within which we can be 95% sure that the true population value lies. Note that the remaining 5% of the time, the value may fall outside this interval. The estimate, which is the effect size observed in the particular study, is the point at which the true value is most likely to fall, though it can theoretically occur at any point within the confidence interval (or even outside it, as just alluded to).

Example

A study is conducted to estimate the average glucose levels in patients admitted with diabetic ketoacidosis. Samples of 100 patients were selected and the mean was found to be 500 mg/dL with a 95% confidence interval of 320-780. This means that there is a 95% chance that the true mean of all patients will lie between 320 and 780.

Hypothesis Testing

Setting up the hypotheses: The basic concept used in hypothesis testing is that it is far easier to show that something is false than to prove that it is true.

Two mutually exclusive and competing hypotheses

Let us consider a situation where we want to test if a new drug is having superior efficacy to one of the standard drugs prevailing in the market for the treatment of tuberculosis. We will have to construct a null hypothesis and alternative hypothesis for this experiment as below:

1. The "null" hypothesis (H0)

The null hypothesis indicates a neutral position (or the status quo in an interventional trial) in the given study or experiment. Typically the investigator hopes to prove this hypothesis wrong so that the alternate hypothesis, which encompasses the concept of interest to the investigator, can be accepted.

Example: In the situation given above, though we actually want to prove the new drug to be effective, we should proceed with a neutral attitude while doing the experiment so our null hypothesis will be stated as follows:

Ho: *There is no difference between the effect of new drug and standard drug in treating tuberculosis*

2. The "alternative" hypothesis (H1)

This is the hypothesis we believe or hope is true.

Example: In the above situation if we want to prove the new drug is superior then our alternative hypothesis will be:

H_1: *New drug's effect is superior to that of the standard drug.*

Based on the alternative hypothesis the test will become one-tailed test or two-tailed test. Two-tailed tests are done when the researcher wants to test in both the directions for the population parameter specified in the null hypothesis (i.e. either greater or lesser). If he wants to test the parameter of the null hypothesis in only one direction (greater or lesser), it becomes a one-tailed test.

In the above example, the researcher test framed the alternative hypothesis in only one direction (new drug is superior to the standard drug) so the test becomes a one-tailed test.

b. Selecting a "significance level" (α)

Significance level is the probability of rejecting the null hypothesis when it is actually true (Type I error). It is usually set at 5%, i.e., a = 0.05 (5%)

c. Calculating the test statistics and p value

Test statistics: Calculating the test statistics will depend on our null hypothesis. It may be testing a single mean or proportion or it may be comparing two means or proportions.

p-value: A p-value gives the likelihood of the study effect, given that the null hypothesis is true. For example, a p-value of .03 means that, assuming that the treatment has no effect, and given the sample size, **an effect as large as the observed effect** would be seen in only 3% of studies.

In other words it gives the chance of observing a difference (effect) from the sample when the null hypothesis is true. For example, if we get a p value of 0.02, then there is only a 2% chance for observing a difference (effect) from the sample, if we assume that the null hypothesis is true.

The p-value obtained in the study is evaluated against the significance level, alpha. If alpha is set at .05, then a p-value less than .05 is required to reject the null hypothesis and thereby establish statistical significance. Purely by convention (without any particular mathematical dictum), this cut-off has become the accepted scientific practice worldwide and the phrase "p<.05" has thus become firmly entrenched in the medical literature.

d) Decision rule

We can reject H_0 if the p-value $<\alpha$

Most statistical packages calculate the p-value for a 2-tailed test. If we are conducting a 1-tailed test, we must divide the p-value by 2 before deciding whether it is acceptable. (In SPSS output, the p-value is labeled "Sig (2-tailed).")

Table 3.2: Step by step guide to applying hypothesis testing in research

Step No.	Action
1.	Formulate a research question.
2.	Formulate a research/alternative hypothesis.
3.	Formulate the null hypothesis.
4.	Collect data.
5.	Reference a sampling distribution of the particular statistic assuming that H_0 is true (in the cases so far, a sampling distribution of the mean).
6.	Decide on a significance level (α), typically .05.
7.	Compute the appropriate test statistic.
8.	Calculate p value.
9.	Reject H_0, if the p value is less than the set level of significance; otherwise, accept H_0.

Hypothesis Testing for Different Situations

Testing for single mean – large samples: Z-test

Z-test for single mean is useful when we want to test a sample mean against the population mean when the sample size is large (i.e. more than 30).

Example

A researcher wants to test the statement that the mean level of dopamine is greater than 36 in individuals with schizophrenia. He collects a sample of 54 patients with schizophrenia.

The researcher can test the hypothesis using Z-test for testing single mean.

Testing for two means – large samples: Z-test for comparing two means

Z-test for comparing two means is useful when we want to compare two sample means when the sample is size is large (i.e. more than 30).

Example

Past studies show that Indian men have higher cholesterol levels than Indian women. A sample of 100 males and females was taken and their cholesterol levels measured. Males were found to have a mean cholesterol level of 188 mg/dL and females a mean level of 164 mg/dL. Is there sufficient evidence to conclude that the males are indeed having a higher cholesterol level?

Here we can test the hypothesis using Z-test for comparing two sample means.

Testing for single mean – t-test

The t-test for single mean is useful when we want to test a sample mean against the population mean when the sample is size is small (i.e. less than 30).

Example

A researcher wants to test the statement that the mean age of diabetic patients in his district is greater than 60 years. He draws a sample of 25 persons.

Here he can test the hypothesis using t-test for single mean.

Independent sample t-test for two means

The t-test for comparing two means is appropriate when we want to compare two independent sample means and when the sample size is small (i.e. less than 30).

Example

A study was conducted to compare males and females in terms of average years of education with a sample of 9 females and 13 males. It was inferred that males had an average of 17 years of formal education while females had 14. Can it be concluded that males are having a higher degree of education than females within this population?

Here we can test the hypothesis using t-test for comparing two sample means.

Paired t-test for two means

Paired t-test is useful when we want to compare the two sample means when the two sample measurements are taken from the same subject under the study like pre- and post-measurements.

Example

A study was conducted to compare the effect of a drug in treating hypertension by administering it to 20 patients. BP was recorded immediately before and one hour after the drug was given. The question of interest is whether the drug is effective in reducing blood pressure?

A paired t-test can be used for hypothesis testing and comparing two paired sample means.

Testing for single proportion: binomial test for proportion

If we want to test a sample proportion against the population proportion, we can use the binomial test for single proportion.

Example

A random sample of patients is recruited for a clinical study. The researcher wants to establish that the proportion of female patients is not equal to 0.5. The binomial test for proportion is the appropriate statistical method here.

Testing for two proportion: Z-test for two proportions

If we want to compare two sample proportions, we can use the Z-test for two proportions when the sample size is large (i.e. more than 30).

Example

Two types of hypodermic needles, the old type and a new type, are used for giving injections. It is hoped that the new design will lead to less painful injections. The patients are allocated at random to two groups, one to receive the injections using a needle of the old type, the other to receive injections with needles of the new type.

Does the information support the belief that the proportion of patients having severe pain with injections using needles of the old type is greater than the proportion of patients with severe pain in the group getting injections using the new type? Here we can test the hypothesis using Z-test for comparing two sample proportions.

Hypothesis Testing vs. Estimation

- *Similarity:* Both use sample data to infer something about a population.
- *Difference:* Designed to answer different questions

Does a new drug lower cholesterol levels?

Measure cholesterol level of 25 patients before and after administration of the drug — the change in cholesterol is 15 mg/dL (225 before; 210 after)

Hypothesis test: Did the drug alter cholesterol levels?

Yes/no decision. Reject or fail to reject H_0

Estimation: By how much did the drug alter cholesterol levels?

Chi-square Test (X^2)

It is a statistical procedure used to analyze categorical data. We will explore two different types of X^2 tests:

1. One categorical variable: Goodness-of-fit test
2. Two categorical variables: Contingency table analysis

One categorical variable: Goodness-of-fit test

A test for comparing observed frequencies with theoretically predicted frequencies.

Two categorical variables: Contingency table analysis

Definition: It is a statistical procedure used to determine whether the distribution of one categorical variable is contingent on a second categorical variable.

It allows us to see if two categorical variables are independent from each other or are related.

Conceptually, it allows us to check whether two categorical variables are correlated.

Notes

1. If the expected frequencies in the cells are "too small," the χ^2 test may not be valid.
2. A conservative rule is that you should have expected frequencies of at least 5 in all cells

Example

We want to test the association between cancer and smoking habit in 250 patients. The chi-square would be an appropriate test.

Analysis of Variance (ANOVA)

When we want to compare more than two means, we will have to use an analysis of variance test.

Example:

A researcher has assembled three groups of psychology students. He teaches the same topic to each group using three different educational methodologies. The researcher wishes to determine whether the three modalities are giving equivalent results. He tests all the students and records the marks obtained.

An ANOVA analysis can be used to test the hypothesis.

Repeated Measures ANOVA

Repeated measures ANOVA is a useful test when we want to compare more than two sample means and when the sample measurements are taken from the same subjects enrolled in the study.

Example

A trial was conducted to compare the effect of a drug in treating hypertension by administering it to 20 patients. BP was recorded immediately before administration of drug and one, two and four hours after the drug was administered. Is the drug is effective is reducing blood pressure?

Repeated measures ANOVA would be the right way to get an answer.

Parametric versus Non-parametric Tests

Tests that we have discussed, such as the z-test, t-test and ANOVA assume a certain distribution of the variables — typically a normal distribution — and are known as *parametric tests*. Tests that do not make any such assumptions are called *non-parametric or distribution-free tests*.

Parametric techniques are more poweful than non-parametric ones. Non-parametric tests are statistical tests that *do not* involve population parameters and *do not* make assumptions about the shape of the population(s) from which sample(s) originate. These are used in the following circumstances:

• Useful when statistical assumptions have been violated.
• Ideal for nominal (categorical) and ordinal (ranked) data.
• Useful when sample sizes are small (as this is often when assumptions are violated).

Disadvantages of non-parametric tests

Following are some disadvantages of non-parametric/distribution-free tests:

• Tend to be less powerful than their parametric counterparts.
• H_0 and H_1 not as precisely defined.

Non-parametric counterparts of parametric tests

There are nonparametric/distribution-free counterparts to many parametric tests.

• The Mann-Whitney U Test: The nonparametric counterpart of the independent samples t-test.

- The Wilcoxon Signed Rank Test: The nonparametric counterpart of the related samples t-test.
- The Kruskal-Wallis Test: The nonparametric counterpart of one-way ANOVA

Table 3.3: Statistical tests at a glance

Type of variable in the study	Parameters to be tested	Number of variables	Sample size	Test
Ratio variables	Mean	One	>30	Z-test
	Mean	Two	>30	Z-test
	Mean	One	<30	t-test
	Mean	Two	<30	Independent sample t-test
	Mean (same subject)	Two	<30	Paired sample t-test
	Proportion	One		Binomial
	Proportion	Two	>30	z-test
	Mean	More than two	>30	ANOVA
	Mean (same subject)	More than two	>30	Repeated measures ANOVA
Nominal/ Categorical variables	Association	Two or more	-	Chi-square
Ratio variables	Mean	Two	When normality assumption violated	Mann-Whitney test
Ratio variables	Mean (same subject)	Two	When normality assumption violated	Wilcoxon signed rank test
Ratio variables violated	Mean	Moe than Two	When normality assumption	Kruskal Wallis test

Sensitivity and Specificity

Diagnostic tests used in clinical practices have certain operating characteristics. It is important for clinicians to be aware of these test characteristics as they interpret the results of these tests, and also as they determine optimal testing strategies to get to an accurate diagnosis or assign an appropriate prognosis. Sensitivity, specificity, positive predictive value and negative predictive values are key parameters used in the further evaluation of the properties of diagnostic tests. Diagnostic tests are compared to a "gold standard" that is the best single test or a combination of tests that are relevant to the particular diagnosis.

Sensitivity is the chance that the diagnostic test will indicate the presence of disease when the disease is actually present.

Specificity is the chance that the diagnostic disease will indicate the absence of disease when the disease is actually absent.

Positive predictive value is the chance that a positive test result actually means that the disease is present.

Negative predictive value is the chance that a negative test result actually means that the disease is absent.

It is important to bear in mind that sensitivity and specificity depends on the distribution of the positive and negative test results within the diseased and non-diseased populations. Thus, specificity and sensitivity values are independent of disease prevalence. On the other hand, negative and positive predictive values depend on the disease prevalence and pre-test probability. These properties are brought to bear when we consider Bayes' Theorem.

Test	Disease	
	Present	**Absent**
	+	−
Positive	True Positive (TP)	False Positive (FP)
Negative	False Negative (FN)	True Negative (TN)

Sensitivity = TP/(TP +FN)

Specificity = TN/(TN + FP)

PPV = TP/(TP + FP)

NPV = TN/(TN + FN)

Efficiency = (TP + TN)/(TP + FP + FN + TN)

The mnemonics of "Spin" and "Snout" (adapted from those originally suggested by Sackett and colleagues) are extremely useful in remembering the properties of specificity and sensitivity. A highly specific (Sp) test, if positive (p) rules "in" the disease – giving us the mnemonic **Spin**. A highly sensitive (Sn) test, if negative (n) rules "out" the disease – and us the mnemonic **Snout**.

Bayes' theorem

Bayes' theorem states that the predictive value of a diagnostic test will depend on the prevalence of the disease. The positive predictive value for a diagnostic test will thus increase for a high prevalence of disease and decrease for a lower prevalence of disease, whereas the negative predictive value will behave in opposite fashion. Diagnostic tests will thus yield a true positive result more often in a high prevalence population.

ROC curves

ROC curves illustrate the trade-off in sensitivity for specificity. The greater the area under the ROC curve, the better the overall trade-off between sensitivity and specificity. This is a more sophisticated way of determining the optimal points for weighing sensitivity versus specificity, since we know that if one is increased, the other invariably tends to decrease.

Relative Risk (RR)

It is the probability of the disease if the risk factor is present divided by the probability of the disease if the risk factor is absent. Example: A study to evaluate the relationship between a food habit and diabetes might compare a group of people with the specific food habit with a group not on the food habit and follow them for the development of diabetes. If 10% of the people on the food habit developed diabetes and 0.5% of the people not on the food habit develop it, the relative risk would be 20.

- Relative risk of 1: no effect
- Relative risk >1: positive effect
- Relative risk <1: negative effect

Relative risk should be presented with confidence intervals (CI), which to reflect a statistically significant finding, should not contain data points that include an RR of 1. Conversely, it can be seen that if the RR CI *does* include 1, then the RR is not statistically significant.

In the food habit /diabetic example if p value was 0.05 and the 95% confidence interval for the relative risk of 20 was 0.7-25, then statistical significance would not be achieved since the range of values includes 1.

Odds Ratio (OR)

It is similar to relative risk, but is used for case-control studies. The odds of having the risk factor if the disease is present divided by the odds of having the risk factor if the disease is absent gives us the OR.

Likelihood Ratio (LR)

Likelihood ratios are very useful in that they are an indication of the degree to which a test result will change the pre-test probability of disease. LR can be calculated in two ways, one is for a positive result and the other is for a negative result.

For a given test, to get a positive likelihood ratio, the probability of a positive test result if the disease is present is divided by the probability of a positive test result if the disease is absent.

+ LR = sensitivity/(1-specificity)

Probability of a negative test result if the disease is present divided by the probability of a negative test result if the disease is absent gives a negative likelihood ratio.

- LR = (1-sensitivity)/specificity
- LR=1: No effect on pre-test probability
- LR>1: Positive effect
- LR<1: Negative effect
- LR=1-2 or 0.5-1: Minimal effect
- LR=2-5 or 0.2-0.5: Small effect
- LR=5-10 or 0.1-0.2: Moderate effect
- LR>10 or <0.1: Large effect

Statistical Software

The life of medical researchers (and biostatisticians) has been greatly simplified by the ready availability of excellent free as well as commercial software. Commercial software such SAS, SPSS and STATA are widely used while free software such as Epi-info are also extremely useful in statistical analysis. Link for the free statistical packages is given in the recommended resources at the end of this chapter.

Survival Analysis

Survival analysis is a form of time to event analysis. In other words, it is defined as measuring the time between an origin point and an end point, often the end point will be taken as death of the patient, occurrence of symptoms or disease onset in clinical research.

Aims of survival analysis may be to estimate survival, compare survival times between two groups or know the relationship of the explanatory variables with the survival time. Survival analysis involves concepts of *censoring* in estimating the survival times.

Censoring

Censoring is defined as study of incomplete observations of the survival time. The following are the types of censoring used in the survival analysis.

Right censoring: Some individuals may not be observed for the full time to failure, e.g., because of lack of follow-up, drop out from the study or termination of the study.

Interval censoring: This occurs when we do not know the exact time of failure, but rather have data on two time points between which the event occurred.

Left censoring: This occurs when some subjects have a delayed entry into the study.

Methods of Survival Analysis

Kaplan-Meier Curve

This curve is used to estimate the survival time and also interpret and compare the two groups survival times. An example is shown below (Fig. 3.9).

Cox regression model

It is used to assess the relation between the explanatory variables and survival times.

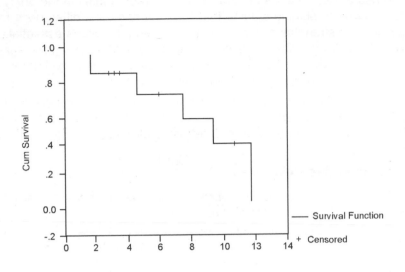

Fig. 3.9. Survival function — Kaplan-Meier curve

Multivariate Analysis

When we want to analyse more than two variables simultaneously we can use multivariate analysis. Multivariate analysis techniques are:

- Multiple Regression
- Multivariate analysis of variance (MANOVA)
- Multivariate analysis of covariance (MANCOVA)
- Canonical correlation analysis
- Discriminant function analysis
- Cluster analysis
- Factor analysis
- Correspondence analysis

Discussing them in detail will be beyond the scope of this chapter. The interested reader can consult the recommended resources for further information.

Meta-analysis

Meta-analysis is used to combine results of similar studies quantitatively to get an overall picture of the problem undertaken for study.

One has to have explicit criteria for inclusion of studies in the analysis to avoid combining studies that have fundamental differences in design. The strengths of meta-analysis is that it functions essentially like a mega-study with increase in sample size and greater generalizability, since data are being captured from studies conducted at multiple sites by differing groups of investigators.

To start a meta-analysis, we will have to identify the articles available related to the problem we have undertaken and then combine the articles which meet our pre-determined inclusion criteria.

Recommended Resources

1. Chatfield C, Collin AJ. Introduction to Multivariate Analysis. 1st ed. London: Chapman and Hall; 1980.
2. Flury B, Riedwyl H. Multivariate Statistics: A Practical Approach. London: Chapman and Hall; 1988. *Hyperstat*, Online at http://davidmlane.m com/hyperstat/Statisticalanalyses.html
3. Sackett DL, Haynes RB, Guyatt GH, Tugwell P. *Clinical Epidemiology: A Basic Science for Clinical Medicine*. 2nd ed. Boston, Mass: Little Brown & Co Inc; 1991.

4

Research Methodology

Ajit N. Babu

■ *What is Research?*

■ *Why do it?*

■ *Basic Concepts*

  ● *Need*

  ● *Science*

  ● *Bias*

  ● *Reliability*

  ● *Validity*

  ● *Causality*

  ● *Statistical Significance*

■ *Ethics*

■ *Research Design*

■ *Getting Started*

■ *Tips on being a*
  Successful Researcher

What is Research?

Definitions abound for research. For our purposes, clinical research can be considered as the systematic process of scientific inquiry to determine etiology, pathophysiology, diagnosis, therapy or prognosis.

Why do it?

The time-honored reason has been to advance the cause of science, enhance our knowledge of disease as well as good health and ultimately lead to the best possible health outcomes for society. Pragmatically, however, there are a variety of personal and professional considerations that lead a medical professional to take up research. It is important to be aware of these different, sometimes conflicting, motivators that underlie modern medical research to fully understand the way that research is performed, appraised and funded.

Individual researchers, in addition to an innate curiosity and desire to contribute to the field, often have practical considerations that encourage them to do research. In Western universities in particular, medical faculty have promotions, tenure and salaries tied to their research productivity. A successful researcher brings in funding to the institution (a process we will examine in more detail later) as well as promoting the academic reputation of the institution by publishing in medical journals and presenting findings at scientific conferences. It can be easily seen by extension why academic institutions also are enthusiastic about research and give pride of place to productive researchers within the ranks of their faculty. However, in developing countries such as India where there is neither an institutional expectation of research by faculty, nor attractive financial incentives, research in academia has tended to be more of a hobby than a science. The winds of global outsourcing that have hit the shores of the developing economies, however, have not left medical research untouched. Indeed, the world is beating a path to these countries for getting clinical trials operational at minimal cost, in settings where significant burden of disease and costs of patient recruitment, research staff salaries and medical care are far lower than in the West.

Basic Concepts

Clinical research must fulfill the following objectives simultaneously (Fig. 4.1):
It should be directed to need.
It should be scientifically sound.
It should minimize risk.
It should be cost-effective

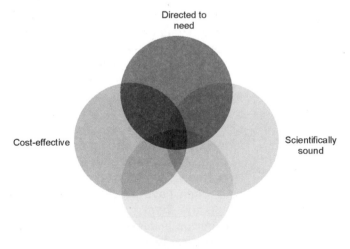

Fig. 4.1. Objectives of clinical research

Research is not easy. Contrary to what the novice might think, coming up with an interesting or worthwhile research question is not the defining moment – rather it is only the beginning. Conceiving and executing the study in successful and even elegant fashion is the real challenge. The first thing is to identify a research question that ideally captures your interest so that you have some intrinsic motivation for plowing ahead even when the going gets tough – and it is fair to say that there will be numerous instances when you may be left wondering what on earth prompted you to embark on such a painful exercise in the first place! Caring about what you are doing will definitely help in such trying moments. Linked closely to this logical concept is that of planning a project that you can reasonably accomplish. A high-powered, multi-centric study with a massive sample size and stellar statistical processes may look seductive on paper, but, by and large, that is precisely where the study will remain – on paper – unless you have the resources to carry out such a grand study (and if you do, then I suspect you don't need to be reading this book!).

Need

First off, sort out a research area in which an answer to the question you are planning will make a difference, a positive one, in the practice or teaching of medicine. After all, if you plan to ask a research question that even you cannot justify as important or meaningful, why should anyone else care (and even worse - fund or publish your study)? The formal approach to this is called a needs assessment. The most practical form of doing it is to look at real-life circumstances (preferably yours) and think about "what needs to be made better" along with a "how". If you can do that, you have the kernel for a meaningful research question.

A more formal way to do it is often through a questionnaire administered to those involved in the actual process you are trying to study or intervene in. For example, if you want to examine the positive effects of introducing an electronic medical record system (EMR) into your outpatient clinic, you will first need to thoroughly understand the current process and get inputs from clinicians, nurses, clerical staff, administrators and other key stake-holders regarding such an intervention via a structured questionnaire.

The next thing is to "avoid re-inventing the wheel", as the saying goes. Why do a laborious study only to find that the same question had already been answered completely by other investigators?

To prevent this embarrassing and frustrating outcome, it is essential to do a **literature survey** to find out the state of the art in the field. Not only will it ensure that your question has relevance, but will also help you to become a content expert in the area, fine tune your study, base it on the state of the art and help avoid elementary mistakes in study conception, design and execution. The wide availability of online databases and the Internet have revolutionized access and analysis of medical information. The downside of this plethora of information is that there is no longer any excuse for ignorance! Chapter 6 provides a detailed survey of available resources and techniques for making the most out of them.

Science

Research at its best is a carefully planned and executed enterprise based upon established scientific principles, not only in its rationale but also in the process followed and outcomes measured. This effort is crafted on best practices in research design. The design selected is ideally the one best suited to the question answered. However, the sophistication of the design will need to be tempered (as in any other sort of undertaking) by the realities of budget, time, administrative considerations and available resources, both human and material. We will examine basic study designs, their rationale as well as strengths and disadvantages starting with the simplest and easiest and work our way up to the more complex. In addition, core principles in design such as bias will be reviewed.

Bias

Bias has been defined by Murphy as "a process at any stage of inference tending to produce results that depart systematically from the true values"[1]. The presence of bias can color research studies at any point and lead to misleading findings. It has been estimated by Sackett that there are 35 different kinds of bias in analytic research[2]. Common examples include selection bias (when comparisons are made of groups that differ in important respects in addition to the main factor being studied), confounding bias (when two or more factors co-exist and the effects of one are modified by the other(s)) and surveillance bias (when one group is studied more carefully than another).

Reliability

This term refers to the reproducibility of a test or measure when performed repeatedly. A highly reliable test, therefore, gives consistent results when used in a setting where the test substrate has remained stable. However, a major part of the final results in many instances is dependant on the opinion of the reader. For example, a chest X-ray is merely an image. Its significance lies in the interpretation of the image by a physician. Reliability in this context can be either intra-observer (which reflects how often the observer reaches the same conclusion in interpreting the same X-ray) or inter-observer (how often two or more observers are in agreement regarding the interpretation of a given X-ray). Since this is a human process, it can be subject to variability and outright error. A statistical measure called the kappa coefficient provides a measure of how great or how little is the variability in the case of nominal data. An alpha of 0 indicates agreement no better than by chance, below 0.40 poor agreement, 0.40-0.59 fair, 0.60-0.75 good, above 0.75 excellent and 1 denotes perfect agreement. The discerning reader by this time may have realized that a reliable measure is not necessarily accurate just because it gives the same result in a given circumstance time after time. Consider a 70 kg man checking his weight on a weighing machine that instead of being correctly zeroed is at the 5 kg mark when not in use. Each time he checks his weight (assuming it remains constant), it will show 75 kg. Highly reliable, but wrong every time! And that brings us to the concept of validity.

Validity

It evaluates whether an instrument or test correctly measures what it sets out to measure. It is immediately apparent that an unreliable measure cannot be a valid one (while the reverse, as we have just discussed, is possible).

Causality

The relationship between something that is responsible for a disease or disorder and the problem itself is causality. It must be kept in mind that just because two or more things are associated, it does not necessarily follow that one is causing the other. For example, let us say you see three motor vehicle accidents near your house. Each of them involves a blue vehicle. From this, though it might superficially seem that perhaps the color blue is a common theme, it would be highly unlikely that the color actually had anything to do with causing any of these unfortunate events.

Statistical Significance

The importance of statistical significance has been covered in more detail in Chapter 3. Here, suffice it to say that a well-designed study will have to be prepared in such a way that it has the ability to demonstrate outcomes that are statistically significant. Results that are statistically insignificant are of questionable value and are typically disregarded by the scientific community.

Ethics

Risk minimization

It is one of the fundamentals of ethical research that the risk to subjects be minimized. There is sometimes a delicate balance between scientific strength of a design and the obligation to protect patients from harm. In case of any doubt, the duty of the investigator (and regulatory bodies) is always to safeguard the patient, even if the science is compromised. This concept has to be borne in mind from the beginning as a research protocol is developed to avoid the need for drastic revisions or even study failure later on.

Research Design

There are a number of established study designs in clinical research that we will now evaluate in further detail, considering in particular the salient features of each, with associated strengths and weaknesses.

Case report/case series

These are essentially publications of the clinical histories of individual patients, either singly (case report) or as a group (case series). It is important to present key information completely and accurately, state what is currently known about the presented disorder or condition and discuss the implications of your report to medical practice at large.

Reports are scientifically justified (and, therefore, potentially publishable) if sharing the findings or observations will be informative to other clinicians and afford new insight into an existing disease or highlight a possible innovation or pitfall in diagnosis or therapy. In olden times before research methodology was well defined, case reports were an important means of communicating possible advances to other clinicians, and many of the seminal findings relating to diagnosis and therapy we take for granted today appeared in print in this fashion.

Case-control (retrospective) study

These are more formal research studies where a group of patients with the disorder of interest are compared to a group without the disorder to see if the exposure of interest varies between the two groups. In clinical research, this is often accomplished by comparing the charts with patients known to have the diagnosis under study (cases) to a group without it (controls). It is ideal to have the cases and controls to be otherwise as similar to each other as possible. However, due to the restrictive nature of this approach where the investigator does not have control over the original data or patient demographics, in practice there can be substantial (sometimes critical) differences that exist between these groups. Compounding the problem, some of these differences may be occult, so that their presence cannot even be adjusted for in the analysis. A better retrospective approach is employed in cross-sectional studies where cases are actually questioned directly (usually via a questionnaire, either administered in person or by mail) about exposures of interest and a selected control group are also asked similar questions. One should be careful not to erroneously classify this approach as a prospective study since the data being collected deals with occurrences in the past, not the future. Cross-sectional studies can only show relationships; these cannot establish causality.

Cohort (prospective) studies

The key feature of these studies is that data are collected from baseline into the future, so that the investigator gets to define the data that is being collected and proceed in a controlled and systematic manner, thereby significantly increasing the quality of the data gathering process. Inclusion and exclusion criteria can also be clearly specified and verified at the time of subject recruitment to ensure adherence to the protocol. Cohort studies often employ the presence of a control group, particularly in case of interventional trials, where the experimental group gets the treatment of interest, and the control group gets either placebo (if ethically acceptable) or standard treatment. After a pre-defined endpoint, typically based either on duration or number of events, the study is analyzed in accordance with statistical procedures outlined in the protocol.

Randomized controlled trials

This is the gold standard for therapeutic trials. It is a cohort study where there is both the presence of a control group as well as one or more intervention groups. Subjects are randomly allocated to these groups at the start of the study in a manner that cannot be influenced by the study investigators. Usually, some sort of computer program underlies the randomization process. The importance of randomization to the study design cannot be over-emphasized. By not deliberately assigning treatments to the subjects, the element of bias can be minimized.

Getting Started

We have discussed so far the theory of research – practically doing it takes planning and method. This is formalized in the form of a research protocol. The protocol contains key elements relating to the research question, rationale, methodology followed, analysis and plan for dissemination as detailed in Table 4.1. In most instances dealing with human research, the protocol and related documentation such as an informed consent form has to be submitted to an institutional oversight committee that is formally charged with reviewing research to ensure that reasonable scientific and ethical standards are maintained within the institution and by their researchers. This committee may be known by different names such as Institutional Review Board (IRB), Scientific Review Committee, or Institutional Ethics Committee. Often, there may be a two-step process where there is initially a review of the scientific merit followed by another committee that focuses on the ethics. The protocol and study documents once approved form the road map for the project. Any proposed deviations from the approved protocol or study documents have to be submitted to the IRB for clearance before the changes can be implemented.

Table 4.1: Components of a human subjects research protocol *

1. Clear research objectives and rationale for undertaking the investigation in human subjects in the light of existing knowledge.

2. Recent curriculum vitae of the investigators indicating qualification and experience.

3. Subject recruitment procedures.

4. Inclusion and exclusion criteria for entry of subjects in the study.

5. Precise description of methodology of the proposed research, including intended dosages of drugs, planned duration of treatment and details of invasive procedures if any.

6. A description of plans to withdraw or withhold standard therapies in the course of research.

7. The plans for statistical analysis of the study.

8. Procedure for seeking and obtaining informed consent with sample of patient information sheet and informed consent forms in English and vernacular languages.

9. Safety of proposed intervention and any drug or vaccine to be tested, including results of relevant laboratory and animal research.

10. For research carrying more than minimal risk, an account of plans to provide medical therapy for such risk or injury or toxicity due to overdosage should be included.

11. Proposed compensation and reimbursement of incidental expenses.

12. Storage and maintenance of all data collected during the trial.

13. Plans for publication of results – positive or negative – while maintaining the privacy and confidentiality of the study participants.

14. A statement on probable ethical issues and steps taken to tackle the same.

15. All other relevant documents related to the study protocol including regulatory clearances.

16. Agreement to comply with national and international GCP protocols for clinical trials.

17. Details of funding agency / sponsors and fund allocation for the proposed work.

---

* Adapted from the **Ethical Guidelines for Biomedical Research on Human Subjects,** Indian Council of Medical Research, 2000

Once the study is ready to commence, one has to identify the appropriate study subjects (or charts in the case of a chart review project). Potential study subjects may be located through advertising (which also usually has to be IRB-approved), word of mouth, referrals from colleagues or personal knowledge. These individuals then have to be evaluated to see if they meet inclusion criteria as defined in the protocol. If so, then the nature of their study and their potential participation in it has to be discussed in simple, unbiased language. Should the prospective subjects be willing to enroll in the study, then they have to sign an informed consent document (unless the need for this has been specifically waived by the IRB). Patient consent is typically not required for retrospective chart review studies, but in countries like the United States, increasingly tough provisions on patient confidentiality may make this mandatory.

Tips on being a Successful Researcher

- Start small–do something that is realistically within your grasp.
- Seek help–from those who are more experienced and knowledgeable than you.
- Do something that truly interests you.
- Develop an area of focus so that over time you can become an expert in the field and develop your career.
- Look for funding–it is a great motivator and enabler.
- Never take dubious shortcuts in the design, process or analysis of your research.
- Get education on research methodology (this book is a small step in the right direction)–many successful researchers have become so by training.

References

1. Murphy EA. *The Logic of Medicine*. Baltimore: Johns Hopkins University Press; 1976.
2. Sackett DL. Bias in analytic research. *J Chronic* Dis. 1979; 32(1-2):51-63.

Recommended Resources

1. Bowling A. *Research Methods in Health*. 2nd ed. Buckingham: Open University Press; 2002.

2.   Fletcher RH, Fletcher SW, Wagner EH. Clinical Epidemiology: The Essentials. 3rd ed. Baltimore: Williams & Wilkins; 1996.

3.   Sackett DL, Haynes RB, Guyatt GH, Tugwell P. *Clinical Epidemiology: A Basic Science for Clinical Medicine.* 2nd ed. Boston, Mass: Little Brown & Co Inc; 1991.

5

An Introduction to Medical Decision-making

James E. Stahl

- Components of Decision

- Choosing Strategies and Framing the Question

- Uncertainty

- Test Characteristics

- Describing Uncertainty

- Values and Tradeoffs

- Interpreting Decision Analyses

- Putting it All Together

We make decisions and judgments every day about every aspect of our lives. Judgment and decision-making are such fundamental human activities that they are often difficult to observe much less analyze. A decision is the process of choosing a course of action in a given situation to achieve a goal. In healthcare, we are often confronted with making choices between competing therapeutic, diagnostic and policy strategies that may significantly influence other people's lives. What often make medical decisions hard are their intrinsic complexity, frequent surrounding uncertainty, frequent competing objectives and frequent critical time-dependence. In medicine, decisions often must be made, good or bad, and not put off. We also must acknowledge that even choosing to observe rather than act is a decision that must be lived with. Therefore, it behooves us to make the best decisions we can. This in turn requires us to examine how we make these decisions.

Decision analysis (DA) and cost-effectiveness analysis (CEA) are quantitative methods for assessing and choosing optimal strategies among many potential alternatives under conditions of uncertainty. These methods involved have been successfully used in a wide array of clinical situations ranging from diagnostic and therapeutic uncertainty, potential therapeutic complications, optimal timing of procedures, and resource allocation[1-6].

Components of Decision

Decisions have structure and are often represented as decision trees in decision analyses. Every decision is composed of at least three components (Fig. 5.1). The first is the set of options or strategies you are choosing among. In a decision tree model, this component is usually represented as the root or decision node. The second component is the set of intermediate events resulting from the chosen strategy. Because decisions take place under conditions of uncertainty, most states or events that occur as a result of any given chosen strategy are best understood as probabilistic events rather than as certainties. This means that in any choice of one strategy over another there is some implicit uncertainty. Events that are governed by random events are represented as chance nodes to the right of the decision node. The third component comprises the outcomes of these strategies and how they are valued. These are usually represented as terminal nodes or health state nodes at the end of the branches of the decision tree. These outcomes must have value; otherwise, there is no real choice to be made. In the healthcare arena, outcomes are usually framed in terms of life expectancy or quality adjusted life expectancy.

Cost-effectiveness analysis (CEA) is the process where two or more strategies are compared with regard to cost and effect. A preferred strategy is one that either provides the same or better effect at either the same or less cost, or one whose incremental cost effectiveness ratio is acceptable[7], i.e., the extra effect is worth the extra cost. Strategies with lower ratios are considered more "cost-effective". Analysis of these models generally proceeds by first determining the best estimates for important parameters in the system in order to perform the "base-case" analysis. Next, the uncertainties surrounding these parameters are estimated, e.g., statistically derived confidence limits. These estimates guide the sensitivity analyses. Here decision models are reexamined while key parameters are systematically varied. These sensitivity analyses allow investigators to understand how the model, and by inference the real system, behaves under various conditions. The choice of parameters to be varied is guided by the hypotheses that they may substantially influence the results. Finally,

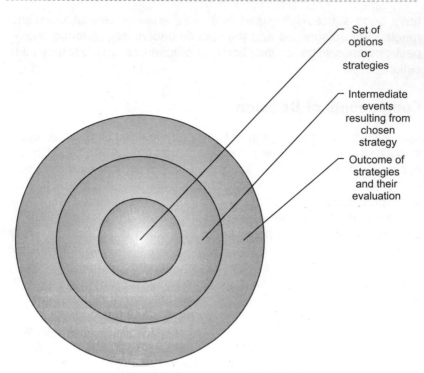

Fig. 5.1. Components of decision

essential to any DA/CEA are utilities - the value people place on an outcome. In healthcare, this is usually framed as quality adjusted life years[7].

Choosing Strategies and Framing the Question

When forming a decision we must choose which strategies or options we wish to compare. This requires understanding the context in which the decision is to be made. For example, are we choosing between medical therapy versus surgical therapy for an individual, or are we choosing how to allocate medical resources for a society? This context defines the range of strategies and options available to us.

We also need to understand who is making the decision and why. All decisions have a perspective from which the decision is taken. Different decision making perspectives – the individual's, a healthcare system's, society's - can lead to different conclusions. For example, giving an expensive therapy, like an organ transplant, to an individual may be correct for that person but may not necessarily be the best answer for society. Perspectives also have consequences in how outcomes are valued and how costs are counted[8,9]. Differing perspectives may also result in conflicts between two or more groups with competing goals.

All healthcare decisions by necessity have an implicit ethical framework. Classic decision analysis starts from a utilitarian perspective[10]. The basic underlying assumption in utilitarianism is that the best decision is the one that maximizes the greatest good for the greatest number of people, or rather maximizes the expected utility of the decision for the population being examined. Using this ethical framework, the strategy that maximizes the number of life-years of a given population should be chosen. This framework has been favored in traditional decision analysis, because it also allows decisions to be articulated in a computationally tractable manner. An alternate ethical framework, often used in medical decision-making, is the Egalitarian/Rawlsian perspective[11]. The underlying assumption here is that the choice that gives the greatest benefit to the worst off person should be given priority. For example, if person A has 1 year to live and person B has 5 years to live and they both would gain 5 years from a given therapy, egalitarianism would suggest allocation of the therapy to person A, who would otherwise die sooner.

It should be noted that people are not completely rational decision makers (as you have no doubt experienced at one time or another!). This influences both the set of strategies and options we consider and how we value outcomes. For example, people make different choices immediately during the event than afterwards, particularly if the decision has significant emotional content, as is often the case in medical decisions[12-14]. People tend to underweigh very high probabilities and overweigh very low probabilities. People tend to value the cost of losing something as greater than the value of winning something[15]. Therefore, while framing our decisions, we must take care to recognize explicitly both our human foibles and values. By being explicit, the validity of our assumptions can be tested and if need be modified.

Uncertainty

Uncertainty is part of every decision. This uncertainty can come from errors in clinical data (history, laboratory, etc.); ambiguity and variations in interpretation, calibration or reporting; relationship between clinical information and disease presence; effects of treatment, etc. To better understand and control uncertainty, we try to characterize it and gather more information. This is where testing becomes so important. Testing is commonly associated with medical decision-making. All clinicians use tests in the course of patient care. A test may be considered any instrument that attempts to sort the world into two or more categories. The history, physical examination and laboratory tests are all different types of tests seeking to sort the world. For example, a blood culture attempts to sort blood samples into groups - infected or not infected. However, diagnostic uncertainty remains a fact of life. As a result, clinicians are always revising their estimate of the likelihood of different diseases in their differential diagnosis as they collect information from the patient and laboratory.

The organizing paradigm for most clinicians is diagnosis, prognosis and therapeusis. We test to establish a diagnosis in patients with signs or symptoms, for example, a culture in a patient with a sore throat. We test to screen for disease among asymptomatic patients, for example, stool tests for occult blood in the general population. We test to provide prognosis, for example, to provide prognostic information in patients with established disease as in a CD4/T-helper count in an asymptomatic HIV-infected person. Finally, we test to aid and monitor therapeusis, for example, to monitor ongoing therapy to maximize effectiveness or minimize side effects as in monitoring prothrombin time in a patient on warfarin. Tests aid decision making by helping to evaluate hypotheses and revise probabilities. Tests add value if they have reassurance value for the patient, help the clinical team know what they are dealing with, identify appropriate therapeutic strategies, avoid inappropriate strategies or help understand the cost-effectiveness of further tests and treatments.

Test Characteristics

All tests have some common characteristics. For example, all tests have a threshold or cut-off value that is used to distinguish one group from another. It is this cut-off that determines the sensitivity and specificity of the test. In other words, a test cut-off determines the proportion of true positives (TP), false positives (FP), true negatives (TN) and false negatives (FN) a test yields in a given population. Sensitivity (or true positive rate) is the proportion of diseased people with a positive test. For example, a throat culture is positive for streptococcus and the patient truly has a streptococcal infection. Specificity (or true negative rate) is the proportion of non-diseased people with a negative test. False negative rate (1-sensitivity) is the proportion of diseased people with a negative test. False positive rate (1-specificity) is the proportion of non-diseased people with a positive test.

In common practice, however, the positive and negative predictive values of a test are more commonly used. Positive predictive value is the proportion of true positive tests out of all positive tests. The negative predictive value is the proportion of true negative tests out of all negative tests.

The underlying reality in which these tests are performed is often referred to as the "prior probability" of disease. This is the "true" incidence of disease in the population being tested. This is important in that the positive predictive value drops rapidly as the prior probability of disease decreases. For this reason, a test that performs well in evaluating patients with signs and symptoms, who have a relatively high prior probability of a disease, may perform quite poorly in a low prior probability screening situation, for example, testing for Chagas' disease in heart failure patients in North America rather than South America. However, negative predictive value often goes up as prior probability of disease drops. This is useful when one wants to rule out disease, for example, testing for a myocardial infarction in a young adult with chest pain.

Both precision and accuracy are also important properties of diagnostic tests. Precision (or reliability) is the ability of the test to get a consistent answer when repeated. Accuracy (or validity) is the ability of the test to get the right answer. It is hard to be accurate without being precise, but it is easy to be precise without being accurate! Consider an example: Let us say a patient has a blood glucose level of 120 mg/dL. It is tested 10 times on a given biochemistry analyzer in quick succession. Each time the value obtained is 200 mg/dL. This reflects a *highly* inaccurate, but *perfectly* precise result...!

Clearly, how often these TP, FP, FN, TN events occur when testing, and the precision and accuracy of the test influence the effectiveness of any therapeutic or policy strategy that relies on the test results, which is almost all, to guide decision-making. More on the fundamentals of bio-statistical techniques in general, and their impact on medical decision making can be found in Chapter 3.

Describing Uncertainty

One of the most important jobs in examining how we make decisions is quantifying and describing uncertainty. Understanding what we know and what we do not and with what level of confidence is critical. The most common description used to describe uncertainty is probability (p). This is the number of ways an event can occur/the total number of possible outcomes. Odds (o) are another way of expressing this likelihood. It is straightforward to convert a probability into odds and vice versa.

To get the odds from probability, simply take the probability and divide it by one minus the probability.

$$\text{Odds} = \frac{\text{probability}}{(1 - \text{probability})}$$

To go from odds to probability, divide the odds by one plus the odds.

$$\text{Probability} = \frac{\text{odds}}{(1 + \text{odds})}$$

Medical decision making, as stated earlier, is iterative. We are constantly revisiting our decisions and revising them based on new information. We often do this using heuristic tools or rules of thumb. However, a better way is through the use of Bayes' Theorem. Bayes was an English clergyman whose posthumous work provided a straightforward and rigorous way to revise probability estimates in light of new evidence. It states that the current probability (the posterior probability) is proportional to the prior probability times the standardized likelihood.

In the context of diagnostic tests this means that the probability of disease given a positive test

$$= \frac{\text{prevalence} \times \text{sensitivity}}{(\text{prevalence} \times \text{sensitivity}) + \{(1 - \text{prevalence}) \times (1 - \text{specificity})\}}$$

Values and Tradeoffs

The final piece in formal medical decision-making is assessment of the value of the outcomes of a decision strategy. Without value, there is no decision. In healthcare, the most common outcome measures used are life expectancy, quality of life-adjusted life expectancy and cost[16]. Life expectancy is straightforward. It is the number of years left to live predicated on the decision strategy chosen. But what is meant by quality-adjusted life expectancy? It seems intuitive that the value someone might place on a year in good health versus a year with a wasting disease would differ and that the quality of life with a wasting disease is worse. One of the standard measures used to quantify this is called the Quality Adjusted Life Year (QALY) and it is particularly useful in assessing the cost-effectiveness of an intervention, especially in a chronic illness. It attempts to express the relative worth to an individual of differing levels of morbidity and life expectancy. In deriving a QALY, one year of perfect health-life expectancy is denoted to be worth 1, while one year of less than perfect health-life expectancy is valued below 1. The obtained number (utility) is a subjective one based on patient preference and can be calculated by the measures mentioned below. The change in this value from baseline to that with the intervention is determined and the resulting number is called the change in utility. This number is then multiplied by the total duration (in years) of the treatment effect to generate the QALY. For example, say a patient with lung cancer has a baseline quality of life value of 0.5. A new treatment could increase this to 0.7, with the value lasting for 5 years. Thus, the QALY = $(0.7-0.5) \times 5 = 1$ QALY gained.

How does one measure the relative value people place on different states of health as required, for example, in calculating a QALY? The most direct way is to ask them. While different individuals will have different valuations, it is possible to estimate an average value and the upper and lower range associated with a health state, if one asks enough people. The most common tools for assessing the utility of a health state are: rating scales, time trade-off questions and standard gamble questions[9,16]. The simplest is the rating scale. This is a simple utility thermometer ranging 0 to 100 where 0 is death and 100 is perfect health. Subjects are then asked to rank on this scale a given health state, such as hypertension or stroke.

Time trade-off questions attempt to use a willingness-to-pay method to assess how much people value a health state. For example, subjects with an illness such as hypertension may first be asked to estimate their remaining life expectancy. Next, they are asked to consider a hypothetical technology that could permanently return them to perfect health but would decrease their survival. Subjects are then asked to quantify the number of years out of their life expectancy (if any) they would be willing to give up in return for perfect health. The utility value then equals (the number of years of expected life - number of years willing to trade-off)/number of years of expected life.

Standard Reference Gambles force the person to assess the utility of the health state against the standard reference of death (which has an assumed utility of 0). Consider a patient-scenario where a one-time application of a hypothetical technology will cure them of their illness, e.g., hypertension, permanently. When the technology works, they are in perfect health for the rest of their lives. However, if the technology fails they will die immediately. Patients are then asked to estimate the largest probability of death they would be willing to accept to be relieved of their disease. The Standard Reference Gamble is this percentage. For example, if a subject is willing to accept a 75% chance of success to be cured (and a 25% risk of death) their Standard reference gamble utility is 0.75.

However, people often are balancing several axes of value when valuing outcomes. For example, the allocation of organs for transplant might involve balancing attributes such as effectiveness, cost, justice, utility, quality-of-life and clinical urgency. This is where multi-attribute utility (MAU) theory comes in. To generate a multi-attribute utility assessment tool, one creates a series of trade-off questions between all the value axes. The axes are then given relative weight depending on the results of these trade-offs. The axes are then combined to give a single measure. The most widely used MAU tests are the HUI[17], the EuroQOL[18] and the SF-36[19]. The three approaches mentioned above are important to keep in mind when designing a research project that may have a component of assessing the value that patients place on health related quality of life and the relative value or impact of a variety of decisions on circumstances to their individual contexts.

Interpreting Decision Analyses

There is no single criterion by which to judge a decision analysis. However, when reading a published decision analysis the reader should keep in mind several questions: Are the methods sound? Are the results valid? Will the results influence my decision-making?

In the methods section, the underlying assumptions and premises of the analysis should be clearly stated. For example, was a societal or health insurer perspective used in calculating costs and what population was used in the base-case? Whatever be the specific statistical or analytic methods used to synthesize data, they should be transparent and reproducible. The choice of strategies examined and outcomes considered should be comprehensive enough to satisfy an expert in the field and be clearly articulated. The effects of the uncertainty implicit in the evidence should be explored over clinically relevant ranges. Utilities should be derived from a representative population in a systematic and defensible way.

When considering whether or not the decision analysis will influence your practice, you, therefore, need to ask some important

questions: Are the differences between strategies clinically significant? Does the uncertainty surrounding the underlying data negate
the important differences between strategies? Do the decision strategies and outcomes being considered reflect your patient population?

Putting it All Together

Decision analysis is a method for explicitly putting all the separate
component parts of a decision together —the alternative strategies,
the probability of events and the values outcomes — in a way that can
be analyzed systematically[9]. The most common structure used to
synthesize this information is the decision tree. The advantage of
decision analysis is that it is explicit, quantitative and prescriptive. It
forces the decision maker to separate the decision problem into component parts, which are analyzed individually and recombined systematically. The decision maker must marshal evidence and beliefs
about key uncertainties (probabilities) and precisely specify values
placed on outcomes. Finally, it helps guide clinicians in deciding what
they should do so that decisions are consistent with underlying
assessments of the decision problem.

Decision analysis also allows the comparative analysis of alternative courses of action in terms of both their costs and health consequences. This then becomes cost-benefit analysis or cost-effectiveness analysis. Here the key concept is the incremental cost-effectiveness ratio. The cost-effectiveness ratio is the net increase in resource
cost/ net gain in health outcome resulting from a given strategy, for
example, how many additional units of health benefit (life years,
QALYs, lives-saved) might be purchased for each additional unit of
cost. Common cost units are healthcare costs (hospital, procedures,
physician services, drugs, miscellaneous supplies, other), induced
costs and savings resulting from index intervention and follow up, time
costs (to patients, families, caregivers, etc.).[16]

Currently decision analyses can be instantiated into computer
models using decision trees, state-transition semi-Markov models[20],
discrete-event simulation models[21] and other methods. These methods are currently available to the non-expert through commercial software programs and have greatly expanded our ability to explore the
consequences of various decision strategies in detail.

In the end, we must make decisions in healthcare. It is, therefore,
vital for us to understand how we make these decisions, so that we
can provide the best possible service to our patients and society.

References

1. Cuchural C, Levey A, Pauker S. Kidney failure or cancer: should immunosuppression be continued in a transplant patient with malignant melanoma? *MDM.* 1999; 4(82).
2. Pauker S, Kassirer J. Threshold approach to clinical decision making. *NEJM.* 1980; 302: 1109.
3. Pauker S, Kassirer J. Therapeutic decision making: a cost-benefit analysis. *NEJM.* 1975; 293: 229.
4. Plante D. Clinical decision consultation service. *AJM.* 1986; 80: 1169.
5. Hlatky M. Is renal biopsy necessary in adults with nephrotic syndrome? *Lancet.* 1982; 2(8310): 1264-1268.
6. Pauker S. Screening for HIV: can we afford the false positive rate? *NEJM.* 1999; 317: 238.
7. Gold M et al. *Cost-effectiveness in Health and Medicine. 1st ed.* New York: Oxford University Press; 1996.
8. Weinstein MC, Stason WB. Foundations of cost-effectiveness analysis for health and medical practices. *New England Journal of Medicine.* 1977; 296: 716-721.
9. Weinstein M. *Clinical Decision Analysis.* New York: WB Saunders; 1980.
10. Mill J. In: Sher G, ed. *Utilitarianism.* Indianapolis, IN: Hackett Publishing Co; 2001.
11. Rawls J. *A Theory of Justice.* Cambridge: Belknap Press; 1971.
12. Ekman P. *Emotions Revealed.* NY: Henry Holt and Co; 2003.
13. Lowenstein G, Lerner J. The role of effect in decision making. In: Davidson HHGRJ, Scherer KR, eds. *Handbook of Affective Science.* Oxford: Oxford Univ. Press; 2001.
14. Lowenstein G. Out of control: visceral influences on behavior. *Organizational Behavior and Human Decision Processes.* 1996; 65(3): 272-292.
15. Kahneman D, Tversky A. Prospect theory: an analysis of decision under risk. *Econometrica.* 1979; 47: 263-291.
16. Gold MR et al. *Cost-effectiveness in Health and Medicine.* New York: Oxford University Press; 1996, 425.
17. Torrance GW, Goldsmith CH. *Health Utilities Index.* Bethesda, MD: National Institutes of Health; 1996.
18. Kind P. The EuroQoL instrument: an index of health-related quality of life. In: Spilker B, ed. *Quality of Life and Pharmacoeconomics in Clinical Trials.* Philadelphia: Lippincott-Raven; 1996. .
19. Ware JE, Jr., et al. *SF-36 Health Survey: Manual and Interpretation Guide.* Boston: The Health Institute, New England Medical Center; 1993.
20. Beck JR, Pauker SG. The Markov model in medical prognosis. *Medical Decision Making.* 1983; 3: 419-458.
21. Stahl JE, et al. Stroke: Effect of implementing an evaluation and treatment protocol compliant with NINDS recommendations. *Radiology,* 2003; 228(3): 659-68.

6

Sources of Evidence and How to Use Them

Vasumathi Sriganesh

- *What is Evidence?*
- *The Evidence Pyramid*
- *Primary, Secondary and Tertiary Sources of Information*
- *Evaluating Evidence*
- *Organizing Searches*

What is Evidence?

The word "evidence" reminds one of the word "proof". When searching medical literature for information on a topic, we need articles that help us decide on a further course of action. Such articles need to yield "evidence" that some methodology has worked and shown results. Usually, such articles are either studies with significant number of participants in a trial, or a long-term study on a topic, or both. Other evidence yielding papers are those where authors have studied several published and unpublished papers on the topic and have reviewed, analyzed and consolidated them.

The Evidence Pyramid

The "Evidence Pyramid" starts with a broad base and tapers to a narrow point, like a triangle. It depicts the fact that at the broad base, there are a large number of articles, which comprise mainly of theories and basic research. As we move up the triangle, we narrow down to smaller number of larger studies, till we reach an apex where there is high quality research in the form of in-depth reviews and analyses.

The standard Evidence Pyramid described by SUNY Downstate Medical Research Library shows the following sequence, with the best studies at the top and the more fundamental ones coming last[1,2]:

Rank	Type of evidence
1.	Systematic reviews / meta analyses
2.	Randomized controlled double blind trials
3.	Cohort studies
4.	Case control studies
5.	Case series
6.	Case reports
7.	Ideas, editorials, opinions
8.	Animal research
9.	In vitro (test tube) research

In terms of information resources, the librarians at the University of Washington Health Sciences Library have come up with a pyramid where they have listed information resources that cover the kinds of studies represented in the Evidence Pyramid. We will take a look at this pyramid after understanding different information resources that provide evidence.[3]

Primary, Secondary and Tertiary Sources of Information

Librarians will tell you that the best way to understand information resources is by classifying them as primary sources, secondary sources and tertiary sources. Primary sources are the documents themselves – journal articles, book chapters, pamphlets and so on. Secondary sources are those that list primary resources using certain arrangements. Examples are library catalogs, bibliographies and reading lists. Tertiary sources are those that list secondary and / or primary sources. Examples are website directories, other meta-lists, some meta-search engines, etc.

Primary sources

Some of the well-known primary sources are discussed below.

Cochrane database of systematic reviews: The Cochrane Library/collaboration was formed in the early 1990s. **The Cochrane Library** is a collection of databases that contain high-quality, independent evidence for informed healthcare decision-making. Cochrane reviews represent the highest level of evidence on which to base clinical treatment decisions. In addition to Cochrane reviews, **The Cochrane Library** provides other sources of reliable information, from other systematic review abstracts, technology assessments, economic evaluations, and individual clinical trials – all the current evidence in one single environment.[4]

Systematic reviews in the Cochrane Database are compiled using very clear-cut, explicit methodology, with a specific aim to reduce bias. This happens at every step – starting from identification and selection of studies for inclusion, and then their collection and finally the Herculean task of combining data from all of them. It is important to understand that each step is a laborious process. For instance, in order to identify studies, the process includes "hand-searching" or manually searching for publications that are not indexed in any computerized database. Next, the computerized databases have to be searched with high quality search strategies to ensure that no publication is left out.

The second step, which comprises the job of including studies for review and excluding others, has the difficult element of ensuring that there is no bias and that the scope of coverage of studies is carefully applied.

The final and most important part – the "combining and analysis" — calls for subject specialization as well as excellent research abilities. The objective before the reviewers is that they must help the reader in identifying which forms of healthcare work, which do not work, and which are even harmful! A systematic review does not need to contain a statistical synthesis of the results from the included studies.

If the results of the individual studies are combined to produce an overall statistic, this is usually called a meta-analysis. A meta-analysis can also be done without a systematic review, simply by combining the results from more than one trial. However, although such a meta-analysis will have greater mathematical precision than an analysis of any one of the component trials, it will be subject to any biases that arise from the study selection process, and may produce a mathematically precise, but clinically misleading, result.[4]

It is also important to understand that systematic reviews in the Cochrane Library are updated once every two to three years. Each review is a primary document and its revised version is considered as the latest update on the topic. Earlier versions are not available on the website; CD ROM subscribers do have older versions that may be referred to for academic reasons like checking for comparisons between the older and latest versions.

Other systematic reviews: Many journals have articles that are systematic reviews. Almost always, the words systematic review will be mentioned in the title of the article. You can search PubMed for such reviews by formulating a search strategy and adding the following: AND systematic review [ti].

Example: anemia AND erythropoietin AND systematic review [ti]

This means you are searching for the terms anemia and erythropoietin – both appearing in an article — and you want the title of the article to have the words "Systematic review". Unlike Cochrane Reviews, any updated studies of such articles may be published in later issues of the same or different journals. So it is important to always look for the latest available systematic review on a topic and, if required, compare it with any older versions, across different journals.

Journals that include only evidence-based articles: In recent years, several publications have emerged which contain only evidence-based studies. Some of these are:

1. ACP Journal Club
2. Bandolier
3. Clinical Evidence
4. Evidence Based Medicine
5. Evidence Based Mental Health
6. Evidence Based Nursing
7. Journal of Family Practice - POEMS

Other Evidence-based Products

1. Best Evidence
2. Clinical Evidence
3. PEDro – Physiotherapy database

Secondary sources

PubMed: This is one of the most well known medical information resources. It is a database produced by the National Library of Medicine, USA and has bibliography and abstracts (where available) of about 4000 biomedical journals. The database is free to search at **www.pubmed.gov.** There is an area called "Clinical Queries" which allows you to search for evidence, but this author's experience is that this feature is more useful for those in search of a lot of articles for writing a systematic review. For searching evidence for patient care, there are certain strategies that one may use in PubMed. It is important to know some of the features and limits in PubMed. One of the most important things to know is that PubMed has a database called MeSH (Medical Subject Headings). Every reference from every journal is first imported into PubMed and then assigned MeSH terms that *describe* the entire article. Some terms may be simply assigned as MeSH, meaning that the article is about such and such a term; others are assigned as MAJOR, which means that the article has a large focus on such a term.

• *Qualifiers [MeSH] and [MAJOR]:* In the PubMed search box, if you key in Hypertension [MeSH], you will retrieve articles *about hypertension.* Hypertension [MAJOR] will narrow down your search to articles that have a "Major focus" on hypertension.

• Every MeSH term may have one or more subheadings. These describe the aspects of the term. Searching a MeSH term with an appropriate subheading gets you still more focused articles. Examples of subheadings are diagnosis, drug therapy, etiology, etc. Searching for Hypertension/drug therapy [MAJOR] will help you retrieve all articles that have a major coverage of treatment of hypertension.

• MeSH terms may also be special types of studies – Evaluation studies, Cohort studies or Retrospective studies.

• Articles that are special types of publications are also searchable by indicating their publication formats – for example Randomized Controlled Trial, Meta-analysis, Clinical Trial, Controlled Clinical Trial, etc.

• Combine the appropriate study types for each type of evidence. For *treatment* (drug therapy), look for *randomized controlled trials (RCT).* For *etiology,* look for *cohort studies.* For *prognosis* again look for *cohort studies or prospective studies.*

• Remember, "Publication Types" can be chosen from the Limits page of PubMed, or once you have fed in your topic based MeSH terms in the search box, you can simply add AND randomized controlled trial [pt] – pt standing for Publication Type.

• For Diagnosis add the term "Sensitivity and specificity"[MeSH].

• Further narrowing of searches is possible as follows:
   ■ For articles on treatment, in addition to searching for RCTs, look for double blind and/or placebo controlled studies. These are not MeSH terms; you can simply add them as text words.
   ■ For articles on etiology, use the term "risk".

- For articles on diagnosis, add the term "predictive value" to your search.
- For articles on prognosis, look for terms "prospective studies", "treatment outcome", "survival analysis" or "mortality".
- It is important to use Boolean operators AND and OR wisely to narrow or broaden searches.

Some Sample Search Strategies

- Leukemia/diagnosis[MAJOR] AND sensitivity and specificity [MESH]
- Leukemia/diagnosis[MAJOR] AND (sensitivity and specificity [MESH] OR predictive value)
- Hypertension/drug therapy[MAJOR] AND randomized controlled trial[pt]
- Hypertension/drug therapy[MAJOR] AND randomized controlled trial[pt] AND (double blind OR placebo)
- Asthma/etiology[MAJOR] AND cohort studies[MeSH]
- Asthma/etiology[MAJOR] AND risk AND cohort studies[MeSH]
- Breast neoplasms[MAJOR] AND prognosis[mh] AND treatment outcome[MeSH] AND survival analysis[MeSH] AND mortality[MeSH]
- To study more about strategies, visit the following website:
- http://www.uic.edu/depts/lib/lhsp/resources/filters.shtml

It is a good idea to go through the Online tutorial on searching PubMed (available in the PubMed website); or better still, go through a training program to thoroughly familiarize yourself with the scope of PubMed and its various search strategy possibilities.

Embase: EMBASE (*Excerpta Medica*) is a comprehensive bibliographic database that covers the worldwide literature on biomedical and pharmaceutical fields. It is produced by Elsevier, a well-known publishing house. Embase is searchable at www.embase.com as well as through some other online hosts, but is expensive and can only be accessed through institutional subscriptions.

Biosis: BIOSIS is a bibliographic database covering worldwide research on all biological and biomedical topics. Records contain bibliographic data, indexing information, and abstracts for most references. It is again a paid resource, best accessed through institutional subscriptions. Embase and Biosis are not easily available for use in developing countries.

Tertiary sources

As mentioned above, tertiary sources compile secondary and/or primary resources. Following are some useful tertiary resources.
Directory of evidence-based resources—Netting the Evidence: Netting the Evidence is a set of Directories of sites dealing with evidence-based medicine. This is an initiative of the School of Health and Related Research, University of Sheffield, UK. Netting the Evidence has directories of websites of primary sources of evidence-based journals, and secondary sources, namely, databases. In addition, it also has sites dealing with information on how to appraise literature, organizations dealing with EBM, etc. Netting the Evidence can be accessed at the following website:
http://www.shef.ac.uk/scharr/ir/netting/

Databases

TRIP (Turning Research into Practice) Database and SUMSearch: These are two tertiary search engines. Each of these searches different resources and retrieves answers. They can be accessed at:
● http://www.tripdatabase.com
● http://sumsearch.uthscsa.edu/

The TRIP database searches other sites that provide evidence-based synopses/summaries, guidelines, primary research, etc. In addition, it also searches Medline for articles on treatment, diagnosis, etc.[5]

SUMSearch is another meta-search engine that searches different resources. This database has a special feature. If it finds too many hits at a first level of searching, it executes more restrictive, contingency searches. According to the website, SUMSearch allows the clinician to enter a query one time, and it will then select the best Internet sites to search, format the query for each site, execute contingency searches, and then return a single document to the clinician. SUMSearch removes the burden on the clinician of remembering too many details of searching.[6]

These two meta-search engines have been around since 1997 and 1998 respectively. There do not appear to be any formal studies comparing the two with each other, or comparing either of them with the search facilities of the sources they cover. It appears that if one has to have a high recall, that is, retrieve a thorough coverage of literature, it would be good to comb each resource thoroughly in addition to searching these meta-search engines.

Evaluating Evidence

Evaluating the evidence you retrieve is very important for two fundamental reasons.
- People who write papers are humans and can make mistakes.
- The evidence you find must be relevant in your local context.

The first reason is self-explanatory. To explain relevance in local context, consider this situation – you are working in a Primary Health Centre and you suspect a patient having a rare disease. You happen to have Internet access and search for evidence for proper diagnosis. The best articles tell you to get a Diffusion MRI done. This may be next to impossible at a PHC. In other words it is not really applicable in your local context.

Criteria for evaluating

There are standard criteria for evaluating all types of evidence-based resources.
- Systematic reviews
- Articles on treatment
- Articles on diagnosis
- Articles on etiology
- Articles on prognosis

Websites that give you excellent evaluation criteria as well as additional information are:
- CASP - http://www.phru.nhs.uk/casp/critical_appraisal_tools.htm
- ScHARR Resources—http://www.shef.ac.uk/scharr/ir/units/crita-pp/resources.htm
- Greenhalgh T: How to read a paper - http://www.bmj.com/collec-tions/read.htm

Organizing Searches

For any topic that you are searching, first define your query very clearly in plain English. Use the appropriate keywords and search the TRIP Database and SUMSearch. For common topics like hypertension, you may get enough references through these; but for topics that are relatively rare or for a combination of rare conditions, you may not retrieve much. It is then important to go through all resources that carry evidence summaries and then search sources like PubMed as well.

In PubMed, one must use different search strategies recommended earlier. Once more, I would like to emphasize that some time invested in learning good usage of PubMed will produce long-term rewards. Finally, if you do find a systematic review in the first instance, do check its date of publication. If it is over two to three years old, do look for a fresh one in PubMed or Embase (if you have access). If there is no recent review, then search for other large studies and trials to check if any recommendation or conclusion has changed in the more recent studies.

The last step in evaluation is extremely important – and that is to match the results to the local context. If the results you retrieve from your search suggest treatment or diagnosis or any other activity that is not suitable in your local context for economic or cultural reasons, then you would need to make your own decisions about what your next step would be.

Another decision-making tool is the application of "The Evidence Grid" (Table 6.1). This is based on the fact that practically all research findings are based on their "validity" and on how long the findings have been used , that is, the "Establishment". The grid is self-explanatory and is an excellent guide to follow for both academic research and application in practice.

Table 6.1: The evidence grid*

	Established	Not Established
Valid	Adopt	Further research
Not valid	Exercise caution	Discard

*Courtesy: Dr. Arjun Rajagopalan, Director, Sundaram Medical Foundation, Chennai, India.

Summarizing, it is important to learn search techniques and their importance. There are several online tutorials, but it does make sense to have some hands-on training in this area. It is equally important to get the help of medical librarians who are trained in searching for evidence, when one is searching the literature for a very specific purpose and cannot afford to miss crucial studies. Appraisal is another skill that is best learnt from a good teacher. Both skills with some practice become fairly easy to follow, and with the help of other professionals and colleagues can be of great use both in research and in practice.

References

1. SUNY Downstate Medical Research Library website. The Evidence Pyramid at: http://servers.medlib.hscbklyn.edu/ebm/2100.htm
2. SUNY Downstate Medical Research Library website. A Guide to Research Methods at: http://library.downstate.edu/ebm/2toc.htm
3. Evidence-Based Practice Tools Summary at: http://healthlinks.washington.edu/ebp/ebptools.html
4. The Cochrane Library Website: http://www3.interscience.wiley.com/cgi-bin/mrwhome/106568753/ProductDescriptions.html (Accessed on December 4, 2006)
5. TRIP Database website: http://www.tripdatabase.com/AboutUs/Index.html
6. SUMSearch website: http://sumsearch.uthscsa.edu/details.htm

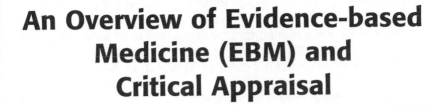

An Overview of Evidence-based Medicine (EBM) and Critical Appraisal

Ajit N. Babu

■ Introduction

■ Components of EBM

  • Defining the problem

  • The Clinical question

  • Finding the evidence

  • Critical appraisal

■ The Evidence-based Medicine Working Group Approach

■ Conclusions

Introduction

The term "evidence-based medicine" (EBM) was coined by Dr. Gordon Guyatt in 1991. He and his associates (led by clinical epidemiologists from McMaster University, notably Dr. David Sackett), formed the evidence-based medicine working group and expanded on this concept in an article published[1] in JAMA in 1992. It was followed by a large series of publications in JAMA spanning over a decade that focused on different elements of EBM. What is perhaps most noteworthy and admirable about the whole movement is that it was essentially repackaging fundamental concepts of clinical epidemiology in a more practical, user-friendly and attractive manner making the principles comprehensible and valuable to frontline clinicians. The EBM movement grew roots across the Atlantic and was strongly supported in England by the NHS and leading universities with major centers like the one at Oxford. EBM has now become a catchword across the globe and the concepts are being applied in diverse settings. Indeed, it would be difficult these days to find any major medical meeting where there was not some presentation or workshop connected to EBM. At the same time, EBM has not been without its critics – some claim that it is a stylized form of cookbook medicine and others allege that it is more hype than substance. Be that as it may, it remains an indisputable fact that EBM is a force to reckon with, and it is important for physicians at all levels to at least be aware of what EBM is, so that they can decide for themselves whether it adds value to their practice, research or teaching.

What is evidence-based medicine?

Evidence-based medicine (EBM) has been hailed as a "new paradigm" by its creators,[1] and defined by Sackett as the "Conscientious, explicit and judicious use of current best evidence in making decisions about the care of individual patients."

Components of EBM

1. Defining the problem

- **What is the clinical issue?**
  It is neither effective nor appropriate to do random searches for evidence as a form of "window-shopping". Time is valuable and if you are going to do an EBM analysis, it is essential to clearly define in your own mind what the clinical issue is, keeping in sight the particular patient whose problem you are working on.

- **Why is it important?**
  Even if there is a well-defined clinical issue, it may not be worth investing the effort to find evidence related to it if the ultimate answer is unimportant, i.e., it does not make a difference to either the patient or the clinician.

- **How will evidence change your management?**
  This is related to the prior question of the importance of the evidence, but has its own implications. For example, consider a patient with advanced, incurable breast cancer. She has no desire for palliative therapy and is aware of her dismal prognosis. In this case, searching for evidence relating to optimal palliative therapy is meaningless and best avoided.

2. The clinical question

It is vital to frame the clinical question in a "searchable" way so that there is a reasonable chance of locating relevant information online. It is rather an art to do it in such a way that the question is specific enough to get you some useful "hits" but not so focused that you miss out on relevant material. A good question has three components: Population-intervention-outcome (can be remembered by the mnemonic PIO). Sometimes, a fourth component can be added – a comparator – making for PICO. Let us look at an example:

In a 65 y/o male with atrial fibrillation, does anticoagulation with Warfarin decrease the risk of stroke?

Here, "65 year old male with atrial fibrillation" denotes the population (this can be reasonably thought of as "elderly males"). "Anticoagulation with Warfarin" is the intervention and "decrease the risk of stroke" is the outcome of interest. Should a comparator be also considered, the question could be reworded as follows:

In a 65 y/o male with atrial fibrillation, does anticoagulation with Warfarin or antiplatelet therapy with aspirin give a greater reduction in the risk of stroke?

3. Finding the evidence

This is the tough part! Clinical research with a strong study design provides the best evidence, and in the case of therapeutic studies, the randomized controlled trial remains the gold standard. Textbooks remain useful sources of basic information and are especially valuable for providing insight into aspects of epidemiology, pathophysiology, clinical features and so on relating to a particular disorder. It is worth remembering though that they are about a year out of date by the time they first appear at the bookstores! Peer-reviewed journals remain the place where original research is first published and debated. It is unfortunate but true that "bad" stuff can get into "good" journals. Thus, merely because an article is published in a famous journal does not necessarily guarantee its quality. The advent of the Internet has opened up a world of online resources both free and paid. For the medical practitioner, probably the most valuable site is PubMed Central, created by the National Library of Medicine, USA. It has extensive archives of full-text articles for 500 major journals, some extending back for over a century. The related site PubMed allows searching for abstracts and linked full-text as well directly from the search page. More about PubMed and other useful resources can be reviewed in Chapter 6. A last resource (no pun intended!) is the time-honored expert. The EBM movement frowns on experts as rendering only opinions and not evidence. However, there is no doubt, as any practicing clinician can attest, that a knowledgeable expert with clinical common sense and a scientific approach can add practical insight into the care of a difficult patient, as well as probably having immediate awareness of helpful articles and newer approaches in his/her field.

4. Critical appraisal

The critical appraisal process forms the heart of EBM. This is where a given article, once identified, is carefully analyzed. Evidence can be of different levels of scientific validity. For example, evidence relating to therapy is graded as shown in Table 7.1, based on the basic design of the study:

Table 7.1: Levels of evidence

Grade	Type of study
A	RCT's
B	Cohort studies
C	Case-control studies
D	Case series and "expert" opinion

Grade A forms the highest level, while D merits the lowest level. A number of factors, in addition to the category of the study, greatly influence the overall nature and credibility of the study. We will examine some of them in more detail below.

4A. Issues in study design

Question, budget, time

It is critical to carefully scrutinize the rationale for the study. Was the study specifically designed to investigate the clinical question under review? Or was the protocol a part of some other, larger, trial that focused primarily on other questions? The latter sort of "piggy-back" trial may be sub-optimally equipped to give an accurate answer to the question you are asking.

Population vs. sample

The population reflects the universe of subjects who have a particular demographic and disease profile. Invariably, since it is impossible to study every single patient who has the disease, investigators recruit a sample, which is a subset of patients from within the larger population that is assumed to reasonably reflect the characteristics of the population. It can be readily appreciated that if the sample is poorly selected, its characteristics can differ in important ways from the population giving rise to erroneous and misleading conclusions.

Power

The power of a study is, simply put, its ability to detect a difference where one exists – for example, in a defined outcome between two groups participating in a cohort study. There are a number of factors that impact on power as discussed in more detail in Chapter 3. In general, the single most important factor in determining power is the size of the sample—the larger the sample, the greater is the power.

Bias

Bias has been defined by Murphy as "a process at any stage of inference tending to produce results that depart systematically from the true values".[2] There are many forms of bias, the more prominent ones being selection bias (groups under study differ in significant determinants of outcome), referral bias (patients coming to a referral hospital typically reflect a sicker, more extreme group compared to the general population) and confounding bias (two factors are associated with one another, and the effect of one is confused with or distorted by the other).[3] There is more on bias in Chapter 9.

Chance

There is always an element of chance in any occurrence. Sound research seeks to minimize the effect of chance, and to also quantify its possible impact on the findings. Tests of statistical significance are designed to serve this purpose.

Internal and external validity

Internal validity refers to the strength of the study and how well its different components fit together. External validity, on the other hand, deals with the generalizability of the study – how far the findings can be extrapolated to settings other than the one in which the study was originally conducted. A study without adequate internal validity cannot be relied upon in any setting, while a study that only has problems with external validity may at least be useful in the particular context in which the study was done. An ideal study would have high degrees of both internal and external validity.

Ethics

The ethical background of the study can never be ignored – indeed it should be carefully scrutinized. An unethical study is never acceptable, no matter how "valid" its findings. More about ethics in research is detailed in Chapter 2.

4B. Sample characteristics

Demographics

Demographics such as age, gender, education, etc. (invariably table 1 in a journal article!) are of great importance in evaluating the true place of a particular study vis-à-vis your clinical practice. For example, a study of diabetes enrolling mainly elderly, Caucasian women in the United States may have only limited relevance in the care of young, Indian males with diabetes. The two important points about demographics, therefore, to keep in mind are:

1. Similarity of the study group to your patient(s)
2. Demographic factors that may have in impact on risk profile, lifestyle patterns, healthcare access, etc.

Co-morbidities

Co-morbidities are the disorders the patient may be afflicted with in addition to the disease of interest. These co-morbidities can play a major role in contributing to the patient's overall clinical condition. Consider a cohort study with two arms, wherein the groups are similar but for the fact that one group has a substantially higher number of smokers. For almost any medical condition one might choose to look at, it is likely that the morbidity and mortality would be greater in the group with a higher prevalence of smokers.

Size

The size of the sample, as alluded to earlier, is a key factor in determining its power. In general, the larger the sample size, the more likely it is to generate statistically significant data with a decreasing likelihood of the apparent findings being the result of chance.

Bias

Bias as detailed earlier is always a threat to the validity of the study, but its presence may be missed in the absence of careful scrutiny.

4C. Statistical significance

Numbers and percentages are often inadequate for assessing the impact of an intervention and so further statistical qualifiers are required to look for statistical significance. An age-old benchmark is whether "$p<.05$". While this can tell us whether the probability of the observed event occurring by chance is below 5 percent or not, it does not give us a measure of the range of the possible effects if the study were to be repeated. The 95% confidence interval tells us the interval within which we are 95% sure the true effect is likely to fall. This gives the clinician much more useful information than a p value, in that the range of possible effects is also shown. The narrower the confidence interval, the higher is likely to be the power of the study.

4D. Patient outcomes

What happened to the patients?

This is, of course, the fundamental question. Typical outcomes include morbidity, mortality, quality of life and functional status.

How was this determined?

It may not be very easy to objectively find out and document what happened to the patients in the study. Certain findings, particularly "soft" endpoints like quality of life have an inescapable component of subjectivity, even when validated questionnaires are used for data gathering. Therefore, one has to balance the conclusions arrived at by the study with an assessment of how robust were the evaluation methodologies for outcome determination.

Was there an appropriate comparison group?

When following a cohort of patients with a disorder over an extended period of time, it is to be expected that they may suffer adverse outcomes due to factors unrelated to the disease of interest. To properly account for the impact of these outside influences, there needs to be a control group that ideally is identical with the target group with the exception of the disease in question. The differences observed in the target group in comparison to the controls would be attributed to the effect of the study disorder.

4E. Clinical significance

Was the outcome meaningful to patients or clinicians?

Clearly, measures like mortality or serious morbidities like loss of limb or permanent loss of function would be meaningful to both patients and clinicians. Other outcomes relating to quality of life may mean much more to patients, while surrogate endpoints that give an insight into the course of a disease and its prognosis may get clinicians excited, but not the patients.

Was the intervention practical?

This is connected to the question of generalizability. Cutting-edge innovations feasible in a tertiary care European center may be completely impossible in a medium level Asian hospital. There is really no point in a clinician spending time reading up on esoteric interventions that she may never be able to offer her patients.

What were the costs and the risks?

The clinical significance of an intervention has to be weighed against the risks to the patient, and the cost incurred both to the patient and the healthcare system. Expensive or risky procedures that carry marginal clinical benefits are unlikely to become a routine part of mainstream medical practice. Remember, statistical significance does **not** equal clinical significance! Statistical significance is a purely mathematical conclusion, while clinical significance weighs statistics, current practice, the patient's overall situation – clinical, emotional, social and financial – and the clinical environment in which care is being delivered. Clinical significance is the ultimate arbitrator of the value of an intervention.

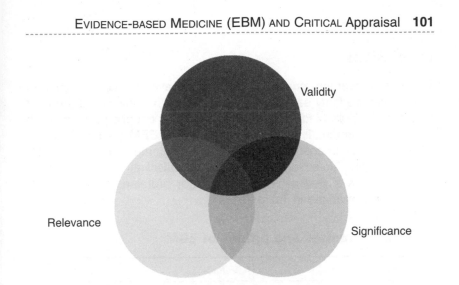

Fig. 7.1. Framework of EBM

5,6. Application and evaluation

This part is relatively simple. Once the evidence has been obtained, apply it and see what happens. If the desired benefit is obtained, well and good. If not, then further review of the evidence is called for to determine an alternative strategy. Should one run out of credible evidence, then clinical judgment comes into play and will hopefully carry the day.

The Evidence-Based Medicine Working Group Approach

The core principles of EBM were initially elucidated by the evidence-based medicine working group in a series of articles published in JAMA which continue to form the foundation of EBM literature. They proposed a fixed framework (Fig. 7.1) for reviewing articles that asked three basic questions with an additional set of primary and secondary questions specific for each category of article. The framework questions are:

1.   Are the results of the study valid?
2.   What were the results?
3.   Will the results help me in caring for my patient?

We will look more closely at this approach in the subsequent chapters dealing with therapy, diagnosis, prognosis and economic evaluation.

Conclusions

The EBM movement continues to bulldoze ahead. The principles of EBM, it can be fairly said, can work for the right clinician, at the right time and the right place. It is worth noting that despite presenting an appealing argument, little evidence shows that EBM is superior to traditional practice in ensuring better patient outcomes. There is universal agreement, however, that critical appraisal is a valuable tool, essential for a skilled clinician. The major promises and pitfalls of EBM are summarized in Table 7.2.

Table 7.2: Promises and pitfalls of EBM

Promises	Pitfalls
More rational, up-to-date care	No time!
Better outcomes	Not enough access to evidence
Higher cost-effectiveness	Many clinical practices (including EBM!) have no good supporting evidence
Growth of critical thinking	Substitutes traditional "expert" with EBM "expert"
Greater physician independence	"Cook-book medicine"?
Greater physician and patient satisfaction	Legal and administrative implications

References

1. Evidence-based Medicine Working Group. Evidence-based medicine: a new approach to teaching the practice of medicine. *JAMA.*. 1992; 268:2420-2425.
2. Murphy EA. *The Logic of Medicine.* Baltimore: Johns Hopkins University Press; 1976.
3. Fletcher RH, Fletcher SW, Wagner EH. *Clinical Epidemiology: The Essentials.* 3rd ed. Baltimore: Williams & Wilkins; 1996.

Recommended Resources

1. Clinicians for the Restoration of Autonomous Practice Writing Group. EBM: unmasking the ugly truth. *BMJ.* 2002; 325:1496-1498.
2. Guyatt GH, Rennie D. Users' guides to the medical literature. JAMA. 1993;270:2096-2097.

3. Oxman AD, Sackett DL, Guyatt GH, for the Evidence-Based Medicine Working Group. Users' guides to the medical literature, I: how to get started. JAMA. 1993;270:2093-2095.

4. Sackett DL, Haynes RB, Guyatt GH, Tugwell P. Clinical Epidemiology: A Basic Science for Clinical Medicine. 2nd ed. Boston, Mass: Little Brown & Co Inc; 1991:145-148.

5. Sackett DL, Straus SE, Richardson WS, et al. *Evidence-Based Medicine: How to Practice and Teach EBM.* Toronto, Ontario: Churchill Livingstone, 1998.

6. Centre for Health Evidence User's Guide to Evidence-based Practice at: http://www.cche.net/usersguides/main.asp

7. eMedicine at:http://www.emedicine.com/

8. JAMA Users' Guides to the Medical Literature at: http://ugi.usersguides. org/usersguides/hg/hh_start.asp

9. PubMed at: http://www.ncbi.nlm.nih.gov/entrez/query.fcgi?db=PubMed

10. PubMed Central at: http://www.pubmedcentral.nih.gov/

8

EBM and Therapy

Ajit N. Babu

■ Introduction

■ The Evidence-based
  Medicine Working Group
  Approach

  ● Are the results of this
    article valid?

  ● What were the
    results?

  ● Will the results help
    me in caring for my
    patients?

Introduction

Clinicians often spend the greatest amount of time pondering over the best therapy, particularly when standard options have failed or not delivered the desired result. Studies of therapeutics are of critical importance and have to be rigorously designed so that misleading conclusions are not arrived at. The most widely accepted standard is that of the randomized controlled trial (RCT). The random allocation of treatments (or placebo) minimizes bias. Further enhancement of the research design is obtained by double blinding – both the patient and the investigator are kept unaware of the nature of the treatment the patient is receiving to eliminate variability in responses or outcomes assessment generated by virtue of knowing whether the patient is getting the experimental treatment or not. There are other research designs, such as non-randomized cohort studies and case-control studies that may also be of value in certain settings as detailed in the research methodology chapter. Non-randomized cohorts are really more appropriate in non-interventional observational trials. When an element of therapy is introduced, the lack of randomization opens up the risk of bias. Case-control studies (also called retrospective studies) have grave flaws and are usually best avoided. However, they have utility in situations where hypothesis generation is the goal or in circumstances where the outcome of interest is rare. In such instances, it may be logistically impossible to mount a large-scale prospective trial. It must be remembered, though, that case-control studies cannot prove causality or evaluate the direct impact of an intervention, which is often the focus of therapy trials.

The Evidence-based Medicine Working Group Approach

Given below are the primary and secondary questions recommended by the working group in their online "Users Guide to Evidence-based Practice" site hosted by the Centre for Health Evidence[1]. More detailed commentary is also available on the JAMA website by free subscription[2]. Both of these are excellent resources and highly recommended to the reader.

I. Are the Results of this Article Valid?

A. Primary guides

1. **Was the assignment of patients to treatment randomized?**
   As discussed at the beginning of this chapter, randomization is the bedrock on which a study of therapy must rest. If the study was not randomized, it will generate much weaker data, and there is an ever-present risk of outright error.

2. Were all the patients who entered the trial properly accounted for and attributed at its conclusion?

a) *Was follow-up complete?*
   Ideally, every patient enrolled in the study should be accounted for when the study is concluded, even if he/she dropped out along the way for one reason or another. If a large number of patients are unaccounted for, it calls into doubt the veracity of the findings. What if the missing patients dropped out because they died prematurely or had significant morbidities? Or, what if they were doing so well that they didn't bother to come back for follow-up? These extreme results are of great importance and losing the patients who have the most dramatic outcomes can clearly lead to misleading conclusions.

b)   *Were patients analyzed in the groups to which they were randomized?*

There are two ways of analyzing patients who are in a cohort trial of therapy: (i) as part of the group they were initially assigned to - an *"intention-to-treat" analysis* (irrespective of whether they actually got the treatment or even crossed over into another group) and (ii) as a part of the group they ultimately ended up in – *an explanatory analysis*[3]. The former is preferred in most cases as it preserves the benefits of randomization and, if anything, is biased against the experimental treatment – that way the risk of inappropriately supporting an unproven therapy is minimized. On the other hand, if there are such a great number of cross-overs that meaningful intention-to-treat analysis is not possible, an exploratory analysis may be better. However, there are significant risks of bias as the factor of randomization has been removed, in essence converting it into a simple cohort trial.[3]

B. Secondary guides

3.   **Were patients, their clinicians and study personnel "blind" to treatment?**

As earlier described, blinding minimizes bias. In therapeutic trials, blinding can be accomplished in relatively straightforward fashion by administering a placebo that is indistinguishable in form, color, taste, etc., from the experimental drug. There are, however, other types of trials where direct blinding is unlikely to be feasible. Consider, for example, a trial looking at conservative therapy versus early surgery for patients with low back pain and disc prolapse. Naturally, it would seem impossible to blind the doctors or the patients to the form of therapy the patient is receiving (However, there have been some creative attempts at doing "sham" procedures to fool patients into believing they were in the intervention group, such as that reported by Moseley et al. on the effects of sham arthroscopy.[4] An interesting editorial by Flum debated the ethical approach of using a similar design for evaluating spinal pain[5]). In such an instance, the problem of bias can be tackled through *blinded outcomes assessment*. This is where the assessor of the defined outcomes is blinded to the therapy that was provided to the group – they are made aware only of the reported outcomes.

4.   **Were the groups similar at the start of the trial?**

A properly randomized study with a large sample size will generally end up with similar patients in each group. However, not all therapeutic trials are large or even randomized. In these latter instances, careful attention has to be paid to the composition of the groups to ensure that they are relatively similar with respect to important prognostic variables so that any observed difference between the groups truly reflects the effect of the intervention rather than that of other factors.

5. **Apart from the experimental intervention, were the groups treated equally?**
   Common sense would tell us that if the experimental and control groups are treated differently in addition to the defined intervention, any observed variation in outcome and prognosis between the groups could be at least partly attributable to the disparity in supportive care. Differences in surveillance and follow-up, or degree of provider attention in the nature of additional counseling or even face to face contact can have an effect on outcome, with the more intensively followed group tending to show apparently better outcomes. This is called *surveillance bias*.

II. What were the Results?

1. **How large was the treatment effect?**
   Instinctively, this is what most clinicians would want to know at the very beginning. The EBM approach, however, emphasizes looking only at high quality results. If the study was poorly done, the results are unlikely to be valid and so their reported effect would be immaterial. But assuming that we have gotten through the first question of validity, a central issue is the apparent benefit of the treatment of interest. The outcomes reported may be figures for mortality, incidence/reduction of markers of disease severity like hospitalization as well as onset, worsening, improvement or resolution of defined morbidities relevant to the disease or treatment under study. These treatment effects can, thus, be reported in a variety of ways utilizing percentages, relative risk or odds ratios. More about the latter modalities can be found in the biostatistics chapter.

2. **How precise was the estimate of treatment effect?**
   The reported value of the treatment effect is known as a point estimate. However, as the name implies, this is only an estimate and, as with any estimate, there is an inherent degree of error. In the clinical literature, the favored approach is to report the 95%

confidence intervals (CI) about the point estimate to give a measure of the likely degree of variation. Let us consider an example. An RCT is performed for 9000 patients with advanced heart failure, divided equally into a control and an intervention group. The control group gets standard therapy alone, while the intervention group gets standard therapy plus the experimental therapy. Note that both groups are getting standard therapy, since it would be unethical to treat control patients with a serious condition like heart failure with placebo alone. The same principle applies to the notion of giving the intervention group only the unproven experimental therapy.

The study design illustrated in the example above is, thus, a common approach in therapy trials, especially for medical conditions that are not minor. Assuming that randomization and blinding procedures are rigorous, an observed difference in outcome with studies of this sort could be reasonably attributed to the effect of the experimental therapy, as that should be only significant difference between the groups. It was found that there was 15% mortality in the control group at the end of one year, while it was only 10% in the experimental group. In this case, the *absolute risk reduction* (ARR) would be derived by subtracting the risk in the experimental group from the control group, 15-10 = 5%. The *relative risk reduction* (RRR), on the other hand, would be obtained by dividing the ARR by baseline risk and multiplying by 100; applying this to our example gives us (5/15) x 100 = 33.3 %. It would be possible to calculate a 95% CI for both the ARR and RRR. If one were to calculate the 95% CI of the ARR in this instance, it will be found to range from 4% to 6%. This is a relatively narrow range, showing that there is little error in the estimate (most likely due to the large size of the studied sample). The oft-quoted p value, on the other hand, does not give us a direct representation of the range of possible effect sizes. However, we can indirectly infer the magnitude of the range from our knowledge that the smaller the p value, the narrower is likely to be the effect size range. More details about confidence intervals and p values are given in the biostatistics chapter.

III. Will the Results help me in Caring for my Patients?

1. Can the results be applied to my patient care?

This focuses on the key issue of generalizability. Even if the study was well done, and the results convincing, the findings may not apply to the patient you are taking care of. If the sort of patients included in the study as well as the setting in which the study was done replicates to a reasonable degree the features of *your* patient and practice environment, then it would be fair to believe that the study results would be useful in your patient care.

2. **Were all clinically important outcomes considered?**
   The term outcome really means the end result of a treatment or intervention. Ultimately, if we are treating patients with diabetes, the final objective is not merely to lower blood sugar, but rather to prevent or at least delay the onset of microvascular complications and end-organ damage. However, to demonstrate improved outcomes of this sort, it may take years of follow-up and large sample sizes. In addition, the day to day clinical practice of the typical clinician is focused on surrogate measures. Again, in diabetes, it may include blood sugar levels, glycosylated hemoglobin levels, serum creatinine, urine microalbumin, lipid profile and so on. These measures are also of clinical utility since there is a body of clinical literature showing that favorably impacting on these values leads to improved outcomes. Still, it must be borne in mind that surrogate measures are *not* the same as outcomes, and one has to be careful before extrapolating findings from surrogate data to actual outcomes. Another angle to consider is that patients may have different perceptions of what is "clinically important". The clinician looks at signs, symptoms and test results. The patient worries about family, job and social status. Thus, even though "tests" are looking stable, if the patient is doing poorly, changes in treatment may be essential. Our care must be focused on what is most important to patients, not just on edicts laid down by textbooks.

3. **Are the likely treatment benefits worth the potential harm and costs?**
   Finally, it has be determined if the treatment is appropriate to administer. Just because it is efficacious from a scientific standpoint does not necessarily mean it is wise to use it. The treatment may be inappropriate if it has significant side effects or is prohibitively expensive. Not surprisingly, these criteria are subjective and depend to a large extent on the beliefs and circumstances of both the treating clinicians as well as the patient. An elderly, conservatively minded patient may be disinclined to pursue aggressive therapies for newly discovered lung cancer, even if there is a chance of therapeutic success. Conversely, a young, affluent businessman with the same diagnosis and stage of progression

may be keen on whatever measures are theoretically possible, even ones that are still in the experimental stage. It takes a compassionate and mature clinician to weigh these diverse factors in a professional, empathetic and non-judgmental way.

References

1. Centre for Health Evidence User's Guide to Evidence-based Practice at: http://www.cche.net/usersguides/prognosis.asp
2. JAMA Users' Guides to the Medical Literature at: http://ugi.usersguides.org/usersguides/hg/hh_start.asp
3. Fletcher RH, Fletcher SW, Wagner EH. *Clinical Epidemiology: The Essentials.* 3rd ed. Baltimore: Williams & Wilkins, 1996.
4. Moseley JB, O'Malley K, Petersen NJ, et al. A controlled trial of arthroscopic surgery for osteoarthritis of the knee. *N Engl J Med.* 2002; 347:81-88.
5. Flum DR. Interpreting surgical trials with subjective outcomes: Avoiding unSPORTsmanlike conduct. *JAMA.* 2006, Nov 22/29; 296:2483-5.

Recommended Resources

1. Evidence-Based Medicine Working Group. Evidence-based medicine: a new approach to teaching the practice of medicine. *JAMA.* 1992;268:2420-2425.
2. Guyatt GH, Rennie D. Users' guides to the medical literature. *JAMA.* 1993;270:2096-2097.
3. Oxman AD, Sackett DL, Guyatt GH, for the Evidence-Based Medicine Working Group. Users' guides to the medical literature, I: how to get started. JAMA. 1993;270:2093-2095.
4. Sackett DL, Haynes RB, Guyatt GH, Tugwell P. *Clinical Epidemiology: A Basic Science for Clinical Medicine.* 2nd ed. Boston, Mass: Little Brown and Co Inc; 1991:145-148.
5. Sackett DL, Straus SE, Richardson WS, et al. *Evidence-Based Medicine: How to Practice and Teach EBM.* Toronto, Ontario: Churchill Livingstone; 1998.

9

EBM and Diagnosis

Steven M. Kymes

- Introduction

- The Evidence-based
  Medicine Working Group
  Approach

  - Are the results valid?
    Primary guides
    Secondary guides

  - What are the results
    Classification of
    results, positive/
    negative predictive
    value and likelihood
    ratios

  - Will the results help
    me in caring for my
    patients?

Introduction

At the most basic level, diagnosis is the process of translating quantitative or qualitative data into a form that allows a clinician to make a "yes" or "no" decision (known in statistical terms as a dichotomous outcome). The yes/no question may take a number of forms: "Does the patient have 'X' condition?", "Should I order an additional test?", "Is the patient's condition worsening?", "Has the patient developed a functional impairment?" Regardless of the question, the answer has a dichotomous form, which mathematically can be represented with "1" (disease present) or "0" (disease absent).

Most clinical data available to clinicians is not in dichotomous form. It is typically continuous (e.g., blood pressure, cholesterol level etc.) or qualitative (e.g., evidence of the presence of adenopathy). Such information does not always easily translate into "yes/no" decisions. Instead, the clinician is required to construct in their mind a model that allows them to convert clinical information into an estimate of the probability of disease. While this is a statistical process, it requires that we ask questions that are the basis of an evidence-based evaluation of the quality of evidence presented.

The Evidence-based Medicine Working Group Approach

The EBM Working Group approach is based on similar analysis of all new information through a common set of questions. These questions force one to examine the (I) validity of results, (II) significance of results and (III) relevance of results to the patient care in a particular setting. Given below are the primary and secondary questions recommended by the working group that present a structured way of critically appraising an article dealing with diagnosis. A detailed review follows each question.

I. Are The Results Valid?

A. Primary guides

The following two questions are the primary guides: (1) "Was there an independent, blind comparison with a reference standard?" and (2) "did the patient sample include an appropriate spectrum of patients to whom the diagnostic test will be applied in clinical practice"?

1. **Was there an independent, blind comparison with a reference standard?**

In performing a diagnostic test, the clinician and patient engage in a game of chance. Like any form of gaming, this is a probabilistic exercise. The patient and physician seek to learn the patient's "true" disease status so they can make decisions regarding treatment. They know there is a procedure that can provide them with perfect information (i.e., the "reference standard" referred to in sub-question #1 above, more commonly referred to in a less precise manner as the "Gold Standard test"). However, the reference standard is typically fraught with risk and expense, so a safer and/or less costly option is often sought. However, in doing this, they must accept that the safer and less costly option (which we refer to as the "index test") will not provide perfect information. Thus, they are left to gamble that the index test will ultimately yield enough information that a decision congruent with the patient's goals can be made.

Consider the following example. Theoretically, we could determine with near absolute certainty whether an asymptomatic man has coronary artery disease (CAD) by subjecting him to a coronary angiogram. This would expose him to significant risks including infection, bleeding, renal failure and local complications. It would also require time off work and thousands of rupees in expense for each procedure. The advantage would be that once the procedure was over, we would know to a near certainty whether the patient had CAD, and assuming he survived the procedure and did not suffer a permanent disability, he might find some satisfaction in that knowledge (his contentment would be somewhat lessened when he is told he will need to undergo the same procedure in two years to ascertain whether heart disease has developed in the interim). The disadvantage, of course, is that he might have to endure significant morbidity or even die as a result of the procedure.

Thankfully, this is not the typical process for screening for CAD. Patients and their physicians do not typically feel that the near-perfect precision of angiography in asymptomatic patients is necessary. Our hypothetical patient and his physician have the benefit of exercise treadmill testing and stress imaging studies to provide a reasonably accurate answer in most instances. However, though none of these modalities subject the patient to the risks and inconvenience of an angiogram, neither is completely accurate in determining whether the patient has CAD. This lack of accuracy is what the patient accepts in return for a safer, less expensive procedure. But in order to quantify this, the patient (and physician) seek an understanding of the degree of inaccuracy that can be characterized as a probability, which is estimated in diagnostic trials.

While the RCT is considered to be the quintessential option for the evaluation of therapeutic interventions, it is not considered to be optimal for evaluation of diagnostic tests.[1] In the evaluation of diagnostic tests, the research question being asked is different than that in therapeutics. When investigating questions relating to therapy, the investigator is seeking to establish causality, while in diagnosis the concern is with correlation (see Fig. 9.1). Correlation is established by comparing the dichotomous decision (i.e., "diseased" or "not diseased") of the observer to the known reference standard (the statistics that are commonly reported are discussed in a later section of this chapter).

In the design of therapeutic trials, measurement of the intervention and the outcome must be independent to ensure an unbiased estimate of effect. Typically, this is accomplished through the use of the "double blind" study design coupled with a blinded (alternatively, "masked") assessment of the primary outcome measure. Properly designed diagnostic trials have similar requirements. In such trials,

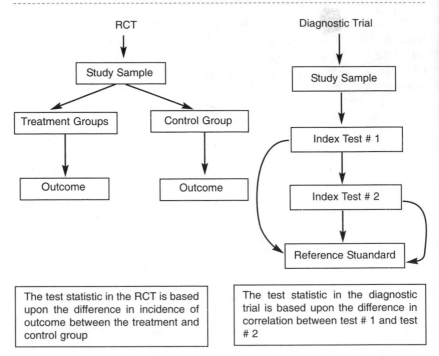

Fig. 9.1. Comparison of randomized clinical and diagnostic trials

the observer translating the results of the index test into a diagnostic decision must be blinded to clinical information unavailable to most clinicians who will use the test in practice — and most importantly, they must also be blinded to results of the reference test. The former is a modest threat to generalizability of the results of the trial. The latter (referred to as "test-review bias")[2-4] is a significant threat to the internal validity of the study.

Consider the following diagnostic trial as an example. A cardiologist who directs an echocardiography lab conducts a retrospective review of the records of 100 people to estimate the accuracy of echocardiography in the diagnosis of coronary artery disease (CAD). She uses coronary angiography as the reference standard. After approval by the Institutional Review Board, she selects the records of consecutive patients from her practice who meet the inclusion criteria and underwent angiography after having echocardiography. In order to avoid bias that may result from her knowledge of pre-test clinical data, she chooses only those patients whose echo was read by her colleagues. She intends to re-read these tests using standardized clinical records prepared by her research assistant.

So far, she has done well. She has avoided the first problem we mentioned. By using standardized clinical records she is ensuring, as much as possible, that she has no more information available to her than the average cardiologist. The threat to external validity is minimized. Yes, we can criticize her for having only one reader, and the as we will discuss in the following section, requirement that the patient undergo angiography is problematic. Still, this is better than most studies seen in the literature. So, now let us assume that she begins her investigation by reviewing the angiography reports of the patients in the assembled sample. Her primary concern, as it would be for any investigator, is that the test was done correctly and the result was recorded accurately in the study records. Having done this, she then turns to reviewing the echocardiography data to assess the index test result.

Our hypothetical investigator has now quite innocently committed test-review bias and seriously compromised the internal validity of her study. She is interpreting the results of the index test with knowledge of the reference test. She has also left the study open to a second threat to internal validity, "Diagnostic review bias", which occurs when the observer interpreting the results of the reference test has knowledge of the result of the index test.[2-4] To most, it would seem self-evident that these violations of blinding should be avoided; however, many justifications can (and have) been offered for the less rigorous approach:

- There is sufficient temporal separation between reviews of the two tests, so it is reasonable to assume that the investigator will not remember the result from one test to the other.
- Identifying headers for the index and reference tests were removed, so the investigator cannot easily link the results of the index and reference tests.
- The investigator attempts to consider only the data presented by the index (or reference) test, when interpreting that test, blocking out any knowledge of the other test to ensure an unbiased result.

These justifications fail to recognize that the knowledgeable reader considering the results of this study when reading a medical journal is not concerned with whether the investigator interpreting the index (or reference) test maintained an unbiased mindset in interpreting the test result. Rather, the reader would be troubled by the fact that there was an element of the study design that was potentially biased, and, therefore, he or she must consider the result of the study as biased. This problem is compounded because the reader cannot know in what direction the bias influenced the result. A recent systematic review of sources of bias identified seven studies that assessed the influence of diagnostic and test review bias and found in some cases it resulted in increased accuracy, on other occasions decreased accuracy was reported, and in yet other circumstances it affected sensitivity and specificity differently.[5]

The defense against these biases is to incorporate features into the study design that *assure independence between the assessment of the index and reference tests.* At minimum, the assessment of the index and reference tests should be conducted by two individuals, each blinded to the other's findings. Larger studies routinely take more extreme measures. For a recent multi-site study of PET in the diagnosis of lung cancer, the PET readings were performed by a panel of readers who were not involved in care of the study participants, at a time and place remote from the patient recruitment and testing. An independent reading such as this virtually eliminates the risk of test review bias.[6] Efforts to eliminate diagnostic review bias were not as rigorous. A local pathologist asked to remain blinded to the imaging result and patient history assessed the reference standard. A superior approach would have been to contract instead with an independent pathology lab to permit the strongest possible blinding to the assessment of the reference standard.[6]

2. Did the patient sample include an appropriate spectrum of patients to whom the diagnostic test will be applied in clinical practice?

In most trials comparing two diagnostic modalities, each study participant acts as his or her own control (see Fig. 9.2). While this eliminates the need for the randomization that protects the internal validity of a clinical trial by reducing the influence of potentially confounding factors, it does make it even more important to address the threat to generalizability (external validity). The primary threat here is referred to as "spectrum bias." External validity of any study is limited by the characteristics of the sample selected. In the case of a therapeutic trial, this bias is referred to as "selection bias." In diagnostic trials, this same form of bias is referred to as "spectrum bias" as it refers to the spectrum of clinical characteristics represented by the patients in the diagnostic trial.[7] Ideally, the trial to establish efficacy or effectiveness should be conducted in a sample that is randomly cho-

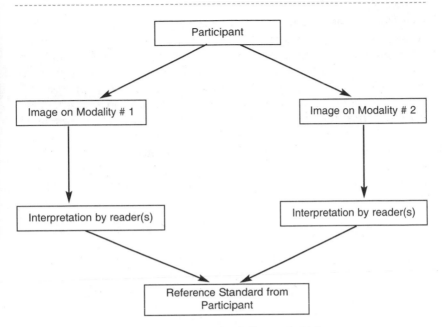

Fig. 9.2. Schematic of diagnostic trial

sen from the population in which the test will be used. This is, however, rarely the case. The accuracy of diagnostic tests is commonly evaluated in diagnostic trials that are conducted in academic or tertiary care settings where there is a high prevalence of disease, but ultimately used more often in community settings where there is a usually a lower prevalence of disease. This bias can have significant impact on the interpretation of results of early diagnostic trials. A study concerning diagnosis of urinary tract infection by use of the urine dipstick found that in patients with severe disease there was a sensitivity of 92%, while patients with a lower pretest probability of disease had a sensitivity of 56%.[8] Thus, a community physician relying on estimates of sensitivity set in an academic setting would vastly overestimate the significance of negative finding on the test. Similarly, early trials of SPECT imaging for diagnosis of coronary artery disease found a much higher result for specificity than was found in later trials and common clinical practice.[9]

An example of this can be seen in studies of the accuracy of PET in the diagnosis of lung cancer. These have traditionally relied on participants with positive or indeterminate results referred from CT. In such studies, the generalizability of PET accuracy would be limited to patients with a higher risk of lung cancer following CT (i.e., PET accuracy would be conditional on a positive or indeterminate CT result). In such a case, spectrum bias would exist if the results were applied to cases referred directly from screening with chest x-ray, or from CT where the patient had a benign finding. Investigators in a recent study of PET addressed this by recruiting participants from a sample of those with a qualifying pulmonary nodule identified on chest x-ray.[6] The consequence of this study design was to increase the proportion of participants in the sample with a benign finding on the reference standard, and to extend the external generalizability of findings to settings where patients have a lower risk of disease.

B. Secondary guides

The secondary guides include the questions: (1) "Did the results of the test being evaluated influence the decision to perform the reference standard?" and (2) "Were the methods for performing the test described in sufficient detail to permit replication"?

1. Did the results of the test being evaluated influence the decision to perform the reference standard?

In all prospective experimental studies (such as clinical trials) or epidemiological studies (such as cohort studies) the decision to conduct the necessary tests to evaluate the study outcome is independent of the exposure. One would not conduct a clinical trial of a glaucoma medication knowing that only the eyes of those who were treated would be evaluated for nerve damage. Similarly, a cohort study examining the link between childhood cancer and high-tension power lines would be ridiculed if only those who live near power lines would be monitored for the presence of tumors.

However, such a bias, typically referred to as "verification bias" is common in nearly all diagnostic trials[10] due to the expense and invasiveness of most reference standards. Let us return to the example of lung cancer diagnosis. In order to conduct an examination of the accuracy of PET or CT in diagnosis of lung cancer, one must use thoracotomy, fine needle aspiration biopsy, or other similar procedure as the reference standard. However, these procedures involve considerable risk and expense. Thus, it would be difficult to ethically justify exposure of participants to these invasive procedures without considerable clinical evidence of the need for such risk. Typically, such evidence only comes from the index test.

Authors have given "verification bias" a number of labels. Some have referred to verification bias as work-up bias or sequential-ordering bias,[7,11,12] while others have suggested that it is a particular variety of work-up bias.[13] Recently, others have sought to distinguish between ignorable and non-ignorable verification bias.[14] In our discussion, we will adopt the following meaning for verification bias:

[*Verification bias*]...occurs when patients with positive (or negative) test results are preferentially referred for the gold standard procedure after which the sensitivity and specificity are calculated only based on those cases who underwent the gold [reference] standard procedure.[13]

As we continue these discussions, it is important to remember that verification bias can be reduced by study design or adjusted for statistically, but realistically cannot be eliminated from diagnostic trials.

To illustrate, let us return to our hypothetical cardiologist. In an effort to make sure that her reference standard is immaculate, she selected only those patients for whom she had a well-defined angiography result. Intuitively, this may seem obvious; however, such precautions limit the generalizability of findings. Echocardiography is performed on patients with a wide range of disease risk—-those referred to angiography for further diagnosis and those who are not. In excluding from the study those who are not referred for the reference standard test, we create a threat to external validity. The consequence of this exclusion is to overestimate sensitivity and underestimate specificity. Shaw and Pryor[15] showed that this bias can be rather severe, resulting in an estimate of sensitivity or specificity that varies from the "true" population based estimate by as much as 20 percentage points.

Many have used a description of verification bias in which it is considered to be present when referral to the reference test is dependent upon the index test result.[16] However, this is a very limited definition of verification bias. Prospective trials can easily be designed in which referral to the reference standard is not dependent upon the index test result, but the trial may still may suffer from verification bias. For instance, assume that we are conducting a trial to estimate the diagnostic accuracy of CT imaging. Our reference standard will be definitive diagnosis based upon tissue biopsy, either surgical or percutaneous. We require that all patients upon enrollment agree to undergo both CT and biopsy, and all those who enroll do. By the definition above, it may seem that we have eliminated verification bias, but that is not actually the case. It is likely that patients with a lower risk of disease will either not be asked to join the study (as the investigator seeks to avoid exposing them to risk of an invasive procedure with no clinical benefit) or the patient declines to participate in a study that will expose him or her to risk and discomfort without sufficient reason.

Simply uncoupling eligibility for the reference test from the index test result is not sufficient to avoid verification bias. The best method to reduce verification bias is through study design. Verification bias is an issue when the disease status of patients with a low risk of disease is not verified because they are not enrolled in the study or are enrolled in the study, but decline to undergo the reference test (i.e., are "lost to follow-up"). If an acceptable alternative reference standard can be established for patients with a lower risk of disease, they might be included in the study, and verification bias reduced. In many studies, a long-term follow-up with the patient to evaluate changes in disease status has been used. In the classic PIOPED study of pulmonary embolism, patients who did not have angiography were followed at regular intervals for a year to assess relevant events.[17] A study of breast cancer followed participants who did not have biopsy for a year to determine if there was any change in breast characteristics.[18] In a study of the accuracy of PET in the diagnosis of lung cancer, participants who did not have biopsy were followed for two years, with those who did not have a change in the size of the solitary pulmonary nodule of interest being considered to have benign disease.[6]

2. Were the methods for performing the test described in sufficient detail to permit replication?

It is a fundamental principle in science that in any scientific experiment, the validity of the results is linked to the extent to which it can be duplicated.[19] This is similarly important when determining the degree to which the results of a diagnostic trial will be applicable to other clinical settings. Specifically, the reader should be concerned with how similar the patients on whom the test was conducted are similar to those in the new setting, how similar the equipment used is to that in the new setting, and the positivity standards employed for the index and reference tests. The space requirements of most academic journals make it difficult to fully present this information. Where it is not found in the primary study report, it might be found in study design papers of larger studies (see Kymes et al[6] for an example of a such a paper), or by contacting the corresponding author of the report.

II. What are the Results?

The question to be asked here is: are likelihood ratios for the test presented, or data necessary for their calculation provided?

Are likelihood ratios for the test presented, or data necessary for their calculation provided? Estimation of the accuracy of a diagnostic test begins with a 2 x 2 table (Table 9.1) to classify the results according to the index test result and the patient's disease status (as determined by the reference standard):

Table 9.1: 2 x 2 Table of test results

Reference Test		+	−
Index Test Result	+	TP	FP
	−	FN	TN

Note that in the above example, we do not consider indeterminate results from the index test. This is not an unrealistic manner in which to consider such a finding. Depending on the consequences associated with misdiagnosis a clinician will consider an indeterminate result either as evidence of disease (and continue the disease work-up or move to treatment) or benign (with the patients undergoing "watchful waiting").

In the 2 x 2 table, TP, FP, FN, and FP refer to true positive, false positive, false negative and false positive results, respectively. From these data, we calculate the primary indices of diagnostic accuracy: sensitivity and specificity[20]:

Sensitivity = TP / (TP + FN)
Specificity = FP / (TN + FP)

Sensitivity represents the probability that a person with the disease will have a positive test result. Specificity represents the probability that a person without the disease will have a negative test result. These are attractive measures to those involved in evaluation of diagnostic tests as they are not sensitive to the prevalence of disease in the population in which the test was conducted. However, these statistics are of little use to clinicians. Sensitivity and specificity begin by assuming that the patient's disease status is known (In the language of Bayesian mathematics, sensitivity and specificity are the accuracy of the test, conditional on the patent's disease status). If the clinician knows the patient's disease status, naturally he or she would not order the test (at least for the purpose of diagnosis).

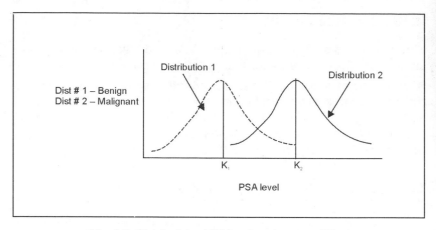

Fig. 9.3. Distribution of PSA values in a population

Sensitivity and specificity have another important limitation that needs to be addressed at length. Consider Fig. 9.3 in which we graph the distribution of a serum disease marker. Let us assume for the purposes of this discussion that the value on the x-axis is the prostate specific antigen (PSA) level in diagnosis of prostate cancer and the y-axis is the number of people with that value. The two distributions (#1 and #2) were constructed by having a qualified pathologist interpret biopsy results from the prostate. On average, people with a malignancy (Distribution #2) have a higher PSA value associated with their tumor than those with benign conditions (Distribution #1). However, there are a substantial number of people with no prostate cancer who have PSA scores higher than some who *do* have cancer.

If we want to know how well the PSA classifies prostatic pathology as benign or malignant, we would to construct a 2 x 2 table similar to Table 9.1 to calculate sensitivity and specificity. To do this, we need to determine what level of PSA we will deem "malignant." In Fig. 9.3, one option would be to use the value at K_1 (which we refer to as our "decision threshold"). We could choose this value because we would achieve 100% sensitivity, correctly characterizing all malignant tumors. But note that at this decision threshold we would also characterize at least ½ of benign tumors as malignant as well (achieving 50% specificity). If this were unacceptable, perhaps we would shift the threshold to K_2 so that we achieve 100% specificity - but now we would incorrectly characterize ½ of malignant tumors as benign (i.e., 50% sensitivity).

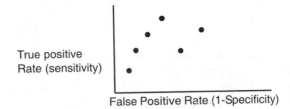

Fig. 9.4. Sensitivity/specificity pairs

This inverse correlation between sensitivity and specificity is characteristic of all diagnostic tests. The degree to which a tradeoff between sensitivity and specificity occurs is a function of several factors, including technical characteristics of the test itself, but it is primarily a function of the variance within the underlying distributions and difference in mean between them. If one were to vary "K" across a range of decision thresholds, the corresponding sensitivity and specificity values could be calculated. We may then wish to examine the relationship between these pairs graphically, so we would graph them in a two-dimensional plane creating a graph similar to Fig. 9.4. By convention, the points are plotted in a plane with sensitivity on the y-axis and 1-specificity on the x-axis. The resulting plane, bounded by 1.0 on both the x- and y-axes is referred to as the ROC space.

If we fit a smooth curve between the points, the result is the "receiver operating characteristic" curve, or more commonly "ROC curve" (see Fig. 9.5). It is a graphic representation of the expected accuracy of the test in a population similar to the sample in which the test was studied.[21] Alternatively, one might consider the ROC curve as representing the possible combinations of sensitivity and specificity that might be achieved with the testing modality.

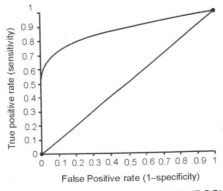

Fig. 9.5. Receiver operating characteristic (ROC) curve

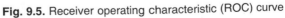

The area bounded by the ROC curve (i.e., the "area under the curve" or AUC) provides an index for comparing the accuracy of diagnostic tests[22]. As an index of accuracy, this is superior to point estimates because it considers all possible decision thresholds, not just a single one. When comparing two diagnostic tests, the test with the largest AUC would be the most accurate, and assuming equal costs of tests, and equal consequences of false positive and negative results, the best possible test to choose is that with the largest AUC[22]. In general, the optimal trade-off between sensitivity and specificity is the point that is at the *top left* of the ROC curve.

Positive/negative predictive value and likelihood ratios

As we have just seen, sensitivity/specificity and ROC curves do not provide clinicians direct evidence that an individual patient has disease. Instead, these methods inform clinicians of the probability, given a patient's disease status, that the index test will yield the "correct" result.[4] However, what the clinician caring for a real patient wants to know is, "If this test gives me a normal (abnormal) result, what is the probability that the patient does not (or does) have disease?" Note that this is precisely the inverse of the information offered by sensitivity and specificity. It should be readily apparent on examining Table 9.1 that this information is contained in the rows of the table (as opposed to the columns on which we based sensitivity and specificity). If we take the row for positive (abnormal) test result, we can calculate the probability of a person having disease by dividing the number of true positives by the total number of positive test results. This is referred to as the "Positive Predictive Value" or PPV of the test:

$$PPV = TP / (TP + FP)$$

Conversely, the probability of a patient with a negative (normal) test result not having disease is calculated by dividing the number of true negatives by the total number of negative test results. This is called the "Negative Predictive Value" or NPV of the test:

$$NPV = TN / (FN + TN)$$

PPV and NPV are often criticized as being sensitive to the prevalence of disease found in the study on which the measure was based. This is not dissimilar to the problems related to spectrum bias which we discussed above, but here the problem is that instead of being an artifact of reader performance, it is inherent in the statistic itself.[4] Consider the following table (Table 9.2) comparing the PPV and NPV that were found in two separate studies, both evaluating the diagnostic accuracy of PET in identifying patients with lung cancer. In the first

Table 9.2: Positive/negative predictive value in two studies with different prevalence of disease

Study #1						Study #2					
Index Test Result	Reference Test +	−	SN	SP	PPV	NPV	Reference Test +	−	SN	SP	PPV	NPV
Positive	188	31	94%	81%	86%	92%	56	6	94%	81%	90%	85%
Negative	12	134					4	23				
Total	200	165					60	29				

. study, patients who were found to have a suspicious nodule on chest radiograph were recruited to the study, and in the second, the patients selected were those that had indeterminate nodules on thoracic CT.[23]

For purposes of this example, we have set the sensitivity and specificity of the two tests at the same level. However, we have not "fixed" the prevalence of disease. In the first study, the prevalence of malignancy was found to be 55% (200/365) and in the second study it was 67% (60/89). In the table we see that even this scant 12-point swing in prevalence resulted in a "flip" of the relationship between PPV and NPV. If the prevalence in the second study were 75%, a level frequently seen in such studies, the result would be a ten-point difference in PPV and NPV between the two studies.

While these differences may seem small, and might even be clinically inconsequential, recall that these differences are seen even though sensitivity and specificity have not changed between the studies. It is strictly a function of the prevalence that is seen in the population in which the study is tested. Given that it is inevitable that the test will be used in a setting where the prevalence of disease is different (most likely less) than the tested setting, PPV and NPV are viewed as less than optimal by most clinical epidemiologists, who advise that they should not be used in reporting diagnostic accuracy or evaluating the presence of disease.[4]

A method that relies on sensitivity and specificity (that is, a measure that is calculated using the column values of the 2 x 2 table) for estimating the patient's probability of disease conditional on the test result would address the limitations of PPV and NPV. This is the purpose of the likelihood ratio. To illustrate how these are used, let us begin by recognizing that every patient who comes to a physician carries with him or her a certain risk of disease. The physician considers the patient's complaints and determines the "pre-test probability" of disease based upon the prevalence of disease among people with similar complaints. For instance, for patients similar to those in Study #1 in Table 9.2, the prevalence of malignancy is 55%. Therefore, if our patient falls into this category, we could say that his or her pre-test probability of disease is also likely to be about 55%. Let us assume that our patient had a positive (abnormal) test result and that the sensitivity of the test is 88% and the specificity, 87%. So, if our patient is diseased, there is an 88% chance that the test would yield a positive result. But what is the probability of getting a positive test result if he (or she) does not have disease? That would be the complement to specificity — 1-0.87, or 13%. Given these probabilities and a positive test result, what would be the odds that the patient is diseased? That would be the ratio of the probability of getting the positive result if the patient has the disease (sensitivity) divided by the probability of getting the positive test result if the patient does not have disease (1-specficity). In the Bayesian world, this ratio is called the likelihood ratio (positive).

Let's apply this ratio to our patient. First we need to estimate the likelihood ratio (positive) for a thoracic PET scan in diagnosing lung cancer:

$$\text{LR+} = 0.88/(1-0.87) = 0.88/0.13 = 6.77$$

In non-mathematical terms, the likelihood ratio of 6.77 means that for each person who has an abnormal test result and does not have lung cancer (i.e., a false positive), there are 6.77 people who have the positive test result and do have lung cancer (i.e., a true positive). Alternatively, we would say that people who have an abnormal result on the test are 6.77 times as likely to have lung cancer compared to those who do not.

As the likelihood ratio is an odds ratio, we need to initially estimate our patient's post-test probability of disease in terms of odds as well so that our comparisons are appropriate. The pre-test odds are determined from the ratio:

Odds of disease = Probability of disease/Probability of no disease

$$\text{LR+} = \frac{\text{Sensitivity of test}}{1 - \text{Specificity of test}}$$

Eq. 1: Likelihood ratio (positive) for diagnostic test

Given that we have estimated the probability of disease already as 55%, we can estimate the odds that our patient has disease as:

Odds of disease = 0.55/0.45=1.22

Now, we can bring together these two pieces of information by multiplying the pre-test odds of disease by the LR+ to get the post-test odds of disease:

1.22 * 6.77 = 8.27

As it is easier to understand, we should convert this back to a probability using a simple formula:

Probability of disease = Odds of disease/(1+Odds of disease)

In the case of the patient before us, this would be:

Probability of disease=8.27/(1+8.27)=0.893

Or, following an abnormal test result, our patient's probability of having lung cancer is 89.3%.

What if our patient had a negative test result? This would be given by dividing the probability of finding a negative test result in someone without the disease (or, 1 − sensitivity) into the probability of finding a negative test result in someone without the disease, which is specificity. So, the likelihood ratio (negative) would be as shown in Eq. 2.

$$LR⎕ = \frac{1 - \text{Sensitivity of test}}{\text{Specificity of test}}$$

Eq. 2: Likelihood ratio (negative) for diagnostic test

Based upon our hypothetical results for PET in diagnosis of lung cancer, this would be:

LR- = (1-0.88)/0.87 = 0.12/0.87 = 0.138

When applied to our hypothetical patient the result is:

1.22 * 0.138 = 0.168

Using our conversion formula, we convert this back to probability:

Probability of disease=0.168/(1+0.168)=0.144

This indicates that after a negative test result, our patient has only a 14.4% probability of having lung cancer. It can be seen that in this particular example, the result of the PET scan will have a significant impact in making our post-test probability of disease either quite high or rather low.

As a general rule of thumb, where the pretest probability ranges from 30 to 70% (a range at which clinical uncertainty typically prevails) an LR+ of 10 or greater is quite likely to *rule in* the disease while an LR- of .10 or lower tends to *rule out* the disease.

III. Will the Results Help Me in Caring for My Patients?

Here one asks the following four questions:

1. Will the reproducibility of the test result and its interpretation be satisfactory in my setting?
2. Are the results applicable to my patient?
3. Will the results change my management?
4. Will the patients be better off as a result of the test?

Now that the clinician has evaluated the quality of the data describing the accuracy of the diagnostic test, calculated measures of accuracy (including likelihood ratios) and estimated pre- and post-test probability of disease — what should be done? After all, what clinician has is a number — one that ranges from 0 to 1. It tells the probability of disease, but it does not tell us whether to treat, or test, or watch, or send the patient home happy after being told by the physician that he/she is well! The contribution by the diagnostic test to the clinical algorithm is a function of the accuracy of the test, but this is only the beginning of the manner in which the efficacy of the test is judged.

Questions III.1 and III.2 relate to generalizability of test results, a question we dealt with in addressing question I.B.2, so we will not belabor that issue here. On the other hand, Fryback and Thornbury considered the latter two issues over a decade ago when they developed a hierarchy of efficacy associated with diagnostic imaging (see Fig. 9.6).[24] Thus far, our discussion has addressed just the first two levels of efficacy that are presented, as the only question being asked concerned the correlation of the test with the gold standard.

Patients do not want to know the correlation coefficient associated with their tests. If they thought about it long enough they would not be even that interested in whether they have a disease! What they want to know is what can be done if they do have a disease. The physician is in a similar situation. He or she wants to know what should be done. Thus, both the patient and physician are concerned with how useful the information is in determining the correct clinical course of action.

These are the questions that are addressed by "Diagnostic Thinking Efficacy" (Level 3 on the hierarchy). At this level, the issue is whether the information provided is compelling enough to affect the therapeutic decision. Translated into the mathematics we have considered thus far, this would imply that the likelihood ratio is large enough (or small enough, in the case of the LR-) to change the post-test probability to such an extent that it would cause the physician and patient to change their treatment decision.

Level/Name	Examples of Measures
Level 1 Technical Efficacy	Resolution of line pairs Gray-scale range Sharpness
Level 2 Diagnostic Accuracy	Predictive value (positive/negative) Sensitivity/Specificity Measures of ROC curve ("Area under the curve")
Level 3 Diagnostic Thinking Accuracy	Number of cases judged "helpful" in making diagnosis Entropy change in diagnosis probability distribution Difference in subjective pre and post-test probability
Level 4 Therapeutic Efficacy	Percentage of times judged helpful in planning treatment Percentage of times avoided unnecessary treatment Percentage of times therapy changed
Level 5 Patient Outcome Efficacy	Percentage of patients whose outcome improved with test Change in quality adjusted life expectancy Cost per QALY saved with new information
Level 6 Societal Efficacy	Cost/Benefit analysis for society Cost/Effectiveness analysis for society

Fig.9.6. Fryback/Thornbury hierarchy for efficacy for diagnostic imaging

As likelihood ratios are a function of the test's sensitivity and specificity, this means that at least one of these measures must be considerably different from 50% if the LR is to be informative. Looking at Equations 1 and 2 above, we can see that if sensitivity and specificity are both near 50%, the LR would be near 1.0, indicating that the test has minimal impact on the post-test probability of disease. It should also be clear that an estimate of sensitivity or specificity less than 50% (as is seen in some screening tests) would also result in an LR that approaches 1.0. In general, to achieve a likelihood ratio of greater than 2.0 for sensitivity greater than 95%, the specificity must be greater than 50%; and if the sensitivity is low (but greater than 50%) the specificity must be greater than 75%. Should the physician seek an even higher LR, such as 4.0 to change the treatment decision, the specificity must be no lower than 76% (assuming a high sensitivity) or less than 88% (assuming low sensitivity).

At Level 4 on the hierarchy, we are asking how often the results of the test, regardless of the likelihood ratio or post-test probability, actually achieved a clinically desirable goal, such as to improve the decision concerning the preferred treatment or avoid unnecessary treatment. This is not only a function of mathematics, but the decision making style of the patient and physician. If the patient or physician is risk-averse and extremely concerned with the possibility of disease occurrence, progression or recurrence, it is likely that aggressive treatment options will be taken regardless of the test results. At the other extreme, if the patent is unconcerned with risk and prefers no treatment, they will be resistant to treatment regardless of test results. In either of these cases, it is questionable whether a test should be done at all.

While there has been considerable research into decision-making styles of physicians and patients, there have been few studies of the influence of diagnostic testing on treatment decisions. A search of the literature in 2005 found only one study concerning the impact of diagnostic decision tests on treatment decisions that had been conducted,[25] and one that was planned but for which the findings had not been reported.[6] However, such studies have great social import. It is rare that the adoption of a new technology leads to obsolescence of an old one,[26] and one can speculate that a major reason for this is the failure on the part of investigators to determine if the proposed test results in incremental information, or simply provides clinicians a "new toy." The failure to consider the impact of new technology has two important consequences: (1) It results in wasteful use of scarce social resources; and (2) It can result in iatrogenic harm to the patient, as he/she is subjected to unnecessary testing and delay in treatment.

The next stage of the hierarchy, Level 5 addresses the issue raised in question III.4 (we will leave discussion of cost-effectiveness, Level 6, for the chapter on EBM and economic analysis). The question whether the patient has improved or will improve should focus not just on clinical factors (i.e., are we controlling the patients hypertension), but on whether the improvement occurs from the patient's perspective.[27] In the United States, as well as other developed nations it is not uncommon for treatment to be given to patients in response to clinical indicators, but without full consultation with the patient and his or her family concerning their preference for curative, maintenance or palliative treatment. This divergence of views between patients and their healthcare providers can lead to troubling circumstances. Perhaps, the most dramatic example of this is seen among end-stage renal disease patients who routinely choose to end their lives by ending long-term dialysis treatment, in spite of being clinically stable.[28]

In general, such contradictions can be avoided if the physician has been open and honest with the patient concerning treatment options. While much of this may seem like common sense or second nature to the thoughtful and compassionate physician, there has developed in recent years a field of medical study that examines methods to improve patients' ability to comprehend the nature of their condition, the consequences of treatment, and their own values concerning these issues. Examples of this can be seen in work done concerning testing for abdominal pain[29] and more recently treatment of cancer.[30] A full discussion of this is beyond the scope of this chapter, but an extensive library of decision aids and information on the development of such aids as well as the standards for them can be found at Ottawa Health Research Institute (http://decisionaid.ohri. ca/decaids.html).

References

1. Valk PE. Randomized controlled trials are not appropriate for imaging technology evaluation. *Journal of Nuclear Medicine*. 2000. **41**(7): 1125-6.

2. Babu AN, Kymes SM, Carpenter Fryer SM. Eponyms and the diagnosis of aortic regurgitation: what says the evidence?[see comment]. *Annals of Internal Medicine*. 2003. **138**(9): 736-42.

3. Jaeschke RZ, Guyatt GH, Sackett DL, Users' guides to the medical literature: III. how to use an article about a diagnostic test: A. are the results of the study valid? *JAMA*. 1994. **271**(5): 389-91.

4. Sox HC, et al. *Medical Decision Making*. 1st ed. Boston: Butterworth-Heinemann; 1988, 406.

5. Whiting P. et al. Sources of variation and bias in studies of diagnostic accuracy: a systematic review. *Annals of Internal Medicine*. 2004. **140**(1): 189-202.

6. Kymes SM, et al. Assessing diagnostic accuracy and the clinical value of positron emission tomography imaging in patients with solitary pulmonary nodules (SNAP). *Clinical Trials*. 2006. **3**(1): 31-42.

7. Ransohoff DF, Feinstein AR. Problems of spectrum and bias in evaluating the efficacy of diagnostic tests. *New England Journal of Medicine*. 1978. **299**(17): 926-30.

8. Lachs MS, et al. Spectrum bias in the evaluation of diagnostic tests: lessons from the rapid dipstick test for urinary tract infection. *Annals of Internal Medicine*. 1992. **117**(2): 135-40.

9. Diamond GA, How accurate is SPECT thallium scintigraphy? *Journal of the American College of Cardiology*. 1990. **16**(4): 1017-21.

10. Reid MC, Lachs MS, Feinstein AR. Use of methodological standards in diagnostic test research: getting better, but still not good. *JAMA*. 1995. **274**(8): 645-51.

11. Diamond GA, Work-up bias (letter). *Journal of Clinical Epidemiology.* 1993. **46**: 207-8.

12. Choi BCK, Sensitivity and specificity of a single diagnostic test in the presence of work-up bias. *Journal of Clinical Epidemiology.* 1992. **45**(6): 581-6.

13. Zhou XH, Obuchowski NA, McClish DK. Statistical methods in diagnostic medicine. In: Balding DJ, et al., ed. *Wiley Series in Probability and Statistics.* 1st ed. New York: John Wiley and Sons, Inc.; 2002.

14. Kosinski AS, Barnhart HX. Accounting for nonignorable verification bias in assessment of diagnostic tests. *Biometrics.* 2003. **59**: 163-71.

15. Shaw LK, Pryor DB. Sensitivity and specificity of the history and physical examination for coronary artery disease (letter, comment). *Annals of Internal Medicine.* 1994. **120**(4): 344-45.

16. Kent DL, et al. Diagnosis of lumbar spinal stenosis in adults: a meta-analysis of the accuracy of CT, MR, and myelography. *AJR.* 1992. **158**: 1135-44.

17. PIOPED Investigators. Value of the ventilation perfusion scan in acute pulmonary embolism: results of the prospective investigation of pulmonary embolism diagnosis (PIOPED). *JAMA.* 1990. **263**: 2753-9.

18. American College of Radiology Imaging Network, *ACRIN 6652. Digital Mammographic Imaging Screening Trial (DMIST) Protocol.* October 27, 2003. American College of Radiology.

19. Kelsey JL, et al. Methods in observational epidemiology. In: Kelsey JL, et al. ed. *Monographs in Epidemiology and Biostatistics*, Vol. 26. New York: Oxford University Press; 1996.

20. Sackett DL, et al. *Clinical Epidemiology: A Basic Science for Clinical Medicine.* 2nd ed. Boston: Little, Brown and Company; 1991: 441.

21. Hanley JA, McNeil BJ, The meaning and use of the area under a. receiver operating characteristic (ROC) curve. *Radiology.* 1982. **143**: 29-36.

22. Metz CE. Basic principles of ROC analysis. *Seminars in Nuclear Medicine.* 1978. **8**(4): 283-98.

23. Lowe VJ, et al. Prospective investigation of positron emission tomography in lung nodules. *Journal of Clinical Oncology.* 1998. **16**(3): 1075-84.

24. Fryback DG, Thornbury JR, The efficacy of diagnostic imaging. *Medical Decision Making.* 1991. **11**(2): 88-94.

25. Tsushima Y, Aoki J, Endo K. Contribution of the diagnostic test to the physician's diagnostic thinking: new method to evaluate the effect. *Academic Radiology.* 2003. **10**(7): 751-5.

26. Eisenberg JM, Ten lessons for evidence-based technology assessment. *JAMA.* 1999. **282**(19): 1865-9.

27. Clancy CM, Eisenberg JM. Outcomes research: measuring the end results of care. *Science.* 1998. **282**(5387): 245-6.
28. Port FK, et al. Discontinuation of dialysis therapy as a cause of death. *American Journal of Nephrology.* 1989. **9**: 145-9.
29. Castro F., et al. Sequential test selection in the analysis of abdominal pain. *Medical Decision Making.* 1996. **16**(2): 178-83.
30. Langer AS. Side effects, quality-of-life issues, and trade-offs: the patient perspective. *Journal of the National Cancer Institute. Monographs.* 2001(30): 125-9.

10

EBM and Prognosis

Ajit N. Babu

- Introduction
- General Markers of Prognosis
- Study Design in Prognosis
- Survival Analysis
- The Evidence-based Medicine Working Group Approach
  - Are the results valid?
  - What are the results?
  - Will the results help me in caring for my patients?

Introduction

The practice of medicine often seems to focus almost exclusively on diagnosis and treatment. Indeed, a commonly asked question by critical thinkers of any intervention or test is "does it change management?" While thoughtful analysis is welcome, it is observed that sometimes clinicians fail to note that predicting the future course of the disease – which is termed *prognosis* — through one or more diagnostic tests can add enormous value to the patient's quality of life and guide optimal long-term management. Even if the disease cannot be cured or controlled, patients and families will often attach great importance to knowing the probable course of events connected to their disorder. There are also clear medical indications for determining prognosis. For example, consider the case of a patient with a myocardial infarction. Once the patient is stabilized and approaching discharge, would further testing with an exercise treadmill be useful? From the standpoint of diagnosis or therapy, it may seem unlikely to add anything since the major diagnosis has already been made, and acute treatment rendered. However, risk-stratification, when appropriate with an exercise treadmill post-MI, is an accepted approach for optimal care of the patient who has not only been diagnosed with CAD, but has also suffered a serious adverse outcome from this disorder.

There are generally two ways in which one can consider prognosis – either viewing the *natural history* of the disorder, which reflects the course without any treatment intervention or the *clinical course* which is the consequence of how the disease behaves when it is under treatment, be it with medications, surgery, radiation or other form of therapy[1]. Clinicians are typically more focused on the latter, since that is where their active intervention comes in.

General Markers of Prognosis

What are some of the standard parameters used to measure prognosis? They can generally be divided into measures studying either morbidity or mortality. It is only of late that medical professionals are recognizing the importance of morbidity reduction. Earlier, if death was delayed, that was regarded as a victory in itself, without much heed to the kind of life the patient was left with. However, particularly in the case of chronic disorders like emphysema or congestive heart failure, there is a substantial component of day-to-day morbidity that patients sometimes fear even more than death. Depending of the circumstances, mortality time-frames can be considered in different ranges – typically in-hospital, 30-day, 6-month, 1-year and 5-year. Five-year mortality is especially important in studies of cancer prognosis. Morbidity measures, on the other hand, may be much more varied, and depend on the particular disorder under study – for example, in studies of coronary artery disease, the frequency of chest pain, dyspnea, days off from work and so on may all be worth including. Some of these symptoms are important in determining *Health Related Quality of Life* (HRQoL). There are specific measures for assessing HRQoL that can be used across disease domains if they are generic (probably the best known example is called the SF-36) or for evaluating patients with a given disorder if disease-specific, such as the Asthma Quality of Life Questionnaire (AQLQ) for patients with asthma.

Study Design in Prognosis

The classic design is that of a cohort study where one or more groups of interest are followed over a period of time, ideally with a control group. The study sample has to be carefully chosen, after which the cohort can be prospectively tracked for the pre-defined duration of the study or till endpoints that trigger study termination are reached. It is also possible to get useful information about prognosis from retrospective studies, especially the nature of risk factors by the study of the differences in exposures between the "cases" (those with the disease) and "controls" (those without the disease). Some common terms used in prognosis studies include response (an improvement that is usually based on pre-defined criteria and may be either complete or partial); remission (when the patient is free of disease for a defined period of time); and recurrence (where the disease has come back after an apparent disease-free interval).

Survival Analysis

The usual method adopted for survival analysis is the Kaplan-Meier survival curve. If the end point is not survival, then a time to event analysis can be done using the same approach with the difference that the end point will be the occurrence of the event instead of mortality[1]. More about these techniques can be found in Chapter 3 that deals with biostatistics.

The Evidence-based Medicine Working Group Approach

Given below are the primary and secondary questions recommended by the working group in their online Users Guide to Evidence-based Practice site hosted by the Centre for Health Evidence[2]. More detailed commentary is also available on the JAMA website by free subscription[3]. Both of these are excellent resources and highly recommended to the reader.

I. Are the Results Valid?

A. Primary guides

1. Was there a representative and well-defined sample of patients at a similar point in the course of the disease?

The reader should evaluate the samples comprising each cohort and see if they are likely to accurately reflect the larger population of patients with the disorder in question. It is also important that the patients in the diseased cohort should have their illness at a comparable stage. Obviously, if the diseased cohort is composed of subjects with varying degrees of disease severity, then their overall clinical course and progress over time will differ, with the sicker patients having worse outcomes.

2. Was follow-up sufficiently long and complete?

Particularly for a study of prognosis, the follow-up period has to be long enough to allow important outcomes to develop. For example, consider a study of patients with newly diagnosed, locally confined prostate cancer, who are being managed through "watchful waiting", i.e., expectant management without active therapeutic intervention. It can often take many years for patients with this degree of prostate cancer to suffer a clinically significant outcome and so following them for one or two years would be quite inadequate to meaningfully study the prognosis of such a cohort. It is also crucial that only a minimal number of patients be lost to follow-up over the defined period of the study. If a substantial number of patients are lost track of with their outcomes being unknown (in essence failing to complete the study), naturally it cannot be determined whether these patients were well, ill or even dead. Why were they not available for follow-up? Did they move? Could they have died? Were they suffering grave complications of the disease? The opportunity for such troubling questions to arise makes the validity of studies where there were large dropout rates highly questionable. On the other hand, if it is clearly recorded why the patients dropped out, and the dropouts were unconnected to the disease process, then there is less of a threat to the validity of the study.

B. Secondary guides

1. Were objective and unbiased outcome criteria used?

Investigators for a prognosis study, just as in studies of therapy or diagnosis, need to identify and define the outcome measures before the commencement of the study. Even something that seems as straightforward to measure as death can be a problem. In the context of countries like India, there are still not comprehensive databases of mortality statistics. Investigators following a cohort over an extended period of time and looking for mortality are thus dependent on maintaining regular contact with the patient, or getting reliable information from relatives. As can be readily imagined, this is not a very robust way of determining an outcome, even one that seems as final as death! When one progresses to considering outcomes that are somewhat subjective (for example, a diagnosis of heart failure) to those that are extremely subjective (such as pain) there can be considerable scope for variability or outright error. Adding to the challenge is the potential for bias in outcome assessment. A sound approach to eliminating this possibility is to blind the individual determining the outcome.

2. Was there adjustment for important prognostic factors?

When comparing the prognosis of two or more groups of patients, it is vital to look carefully to see whether there were fundamental differences in risk/prognostic factors between the groups, and if so, whether this has been adjusted for in the subsequent analysis. Should there be differences that are unadjusted, then the accuracy of the reported conclusions may be tainted. For example, while considering the prognosis of two groups of lung cancer patients where one group has a substantially higher proportion of patients with concomitant diabetes and coronary artery disease, it can logically expected that this group may have a higher overall morbidity and mortality rate, especially when followed out over the standard 5-year period. The analysis should be adjusted for these differences.

II. What Are the Results?

1. How large is the likelihood of the outcome event(s) in a specified period of time?

Once study validity has been determined, the key question (indeed the major reason you would consult an article on prognosis) is to find out likelihood of the outcome within a given period of time. To think back about our earlier example of patients with lung cancer, the outcome question may be structured "What is the likelihood of the typical patient being alive in five years?" In prognosis studies where survival is an outcome variable, it is common to use *survival curves* such as a Kaplan-Meier curve mentioned earlier.

2. How precise are the estimates of likelihood?

As detailed in the chapters on biostatistics as well as in the EBM overview, likelihood estimates are exactly that – estimates. They are never perfectly precise. The degree of imprecision can be best determined by scrutinizing the 95% confidence interval for the estimate –

the narrower or "tighter" the range of the interval, the greater is the precision of the estimate.

III. Will the Results Help Me in Caring for My Patients?

1. Were the study patients similar to my own?

As discussed in the EBM overview chapter, generalizability is an important factor to consider while reviewing a study. Were the patients in the study similar to the patient(s) you are taking care of? If so, the results are likely to be useful and applicable to your patient as well. If not, one has to be very cautious in extrapolating the results since they may not apply to your patient.

2. Will the results lead directly to selecting or avoiding therapy?

Prognostic studies may look at directly improving prognosis by means of an intervention like medical therapy or a surgical procedure. In this case, a positive study, applicable to your patient, may suggest using a similar intervention for your patient. For example, aspirin therapy in a patient following a myocardial infarction can significantly reduce the risk of a recurrent infarction.

3. Are the results useful for reassuring or counseling patients?

The second form of information that has value in managing or evaluating prognosis is data that may not influence the actual prognosis but does help in defining or quantifying it. Information of this sort may still have meaning for both the patient and clinician, since it clarifies the expected course of the disease allowing the patient to plan his/her day-to-day life with some confidence, and the clinician to plan medical management appropriately. There are times when the clinical outlook is grim and hopes of a cure have to be abandoned with the focus being on supportive measures to comfort and alleviate. It may take even more clinical wisdom to know when to stop than it does to actively treat a disorder.

References

1. Fletcher RH, Fletcher SW, Wagner EH. *Clinical Epidemiology: The Essentials.* 3rd ed. Baltimore: Williams & Wilkins; 1996.

2. Centre for Health Evidence User's Guide to Evidence-based Practice at: http://www.cche.net/usersguides/prognosis.asp
3. JAMA Users' Guides to the Medical Literature at: http://ugi.usersguides.org/usersguides/hg/hh_start.asp

Recommended Resources

1. Evidence-Based Medicine Working Group. Evidence-based medicine: a new approach to teaching the practice of medicine. *JAMA.* 1992; 268:2420-2425.
2. Guyatt GH, Rennie D. Users' guides to the medical literature. *JAMA.* 1993; 270:2096-2097.
3. Oxman AD, Sackett DL, Guyatt GH, for the Evidence-Based Medicine Working Group. Users' guides to the medical literature, I: how to get started. *JAMA.* 1993; 270:2093-2095.
4. Sackett DL, Haynes RB, Guyatt GH, Tugwell P. *Clinical Epidemiology: A Basic Science for Clinical Medicine.* 2nd ed. Boston, Mass: Little Brown & Co Inc; 1991:145-148.
5. Sackett DL, Straus SE, Richardson WS, et al. *Evidence-Based Medicine: How to Practice and Teach EBM.* Toronto, Ontario: Churchill Livingstone; 1998.

11

EBM and Economic Analysis

Steven M. Kymes

- *Introduction*
- *The Evidence-based Medicine Working Group Approach*
  - *Are the results valid?*
  - *Economic comparison of healthcare strategies*
  - *Valuation of costs and outcomes*
  - *Allowance for uncertainties*
  - *What were the results?*
  - *Incremental costs and outcomes*
  - *Change in results with allowance for uncertainties*
  - *Will the results help me in caring for my patients?*
  - *Are treatment benefits worth the harms and cost?*
  - *Could my patients expect similar health outcomes?*
  - *Could I expect similar costs?*

Introduction

Financial strains on the healthcare system in the industrialized world caused by an aging population and increasingly expensive technology have led to a growing share of national economic output being devoted to medical care.[1] This trend has spurred an explosion of cost-effectiveness research over the past decade, with a search of Medline conducted in January 2007 finding over 28,000 citations between 1996 and 2006 that include the MESH heading of "cost-benefit" and/or the key word of "cost-effectiveness". Use of economic evaluation as a decision tool to assist policy makers, clinicians and patients in weighing options for allocation of scarce healthcare resources is not new to the medical sciences. Indeed, it has been commonly used in evaluation of health programs for over thirty years, and today it is considered to be *de rigueur* in decision making by health policy makers in most industrialized nations pondering the adoption of new technologies or drugs.[6] In developing nations the role of economic evaluation in considering newer technologies is not as prevalent but the use of these methods to consider public health interventions such as prevention of blindness is common.[3-5]

In general, most work that is done in economic evaluation is at the level of the local or national health authority and thus remote from the individual physician/patient encounter. However, it is not uncommon for the physician to be placed in a position where he/she is acting as an advocate for adoption of a medication or equipment with a formulary board, hospital administration, or regional health authority on behalf of patients and colleagues.[7] Thus, it is useful for physicians to understand the theories and methods employed by cost-effectiveness practitioners. In addition, properly conducted economic evaluation studies can provide physicians information concerning which patients will benefit most from an intervention or what factors will be most influential in the patient deciding whether a treatment is "worth it."[6]

We will begin this discussion by dispensing with some ambiguity in terminology that is commonly seen in descriptions of economic evaluation. The methods we describe here are often referred to in generic terms as "cost-effectiveness analyses". While this may be an accurate description of the goal of the science, it can cause some confusion among practitioners for whom "cost-effectiveness" (as we will see shortly) is a particular method of analysis. Therefore, most practitioners refer to this field of research as "economic evaluation", referring to the application of economic methods in evaluation of health programs.[3]

The Evidence-based Medicine Working Group Approach

The working group has recommended a set of common questions for evaluating articles dealing with economic analysis. These questions allow uniformity of approach and represent a structured way of logically evaluating the articles.[7,27] An in-depth analysis and discussion follows each question.

I. Are the Results Valid?

1. Did the analysis provide a full economic comparison of healthcare strategies?

The purpose of economic evaluation is to determine whether the benefits derived from a particular health program to treat or prevent disease outweigh the costs associated with providing the program. This comparison is made by developing a mathematical model that describes the incidence and/or progression of disease. The model may incorporate data from a single clinical trial or from various sources including epidemiological studies and cost studies to estimate costs and benefits. The model must represent the entire episode of disease for costs and benefits to be estimated properly. For acute illnesses, this may represent but a few months or years; however, as economic evaluation increasingly concerns treatment or prevention of chronic disease, the "episode" will typically be the person's remaining lifetime.

The purpose of economic evaluation is to make a decision as to whether the proposed health program should be adopted. To inform this decision, the policy maker would consider the relationship between costs and benefits using the *incremental cost-effectiveness ratio* (ICER):

(Incremental cost of intervention over current practice) / (Incremental effectiveness of intervention over current practice)

Eq. 11.1: Incremental cost-effectiveness ratio (ICER)

The decision as to whether or not adopt the new technology will depend on the rule the decision maker applies in interpreting the ICER. Note that the cost and effectiveness that are of interest in the ICER are the "incremental" cost on the new program (i.e., how much more the new program costs than the current one) and the "incremental" effectiveness (i.e., how much more effective the new program is compared to the current one). We are not concerned with the overall cost (and effectiveness). We assume that the cost-effectiveness of the current program has been established (otherwise, it would not be adopted).

As we are concerned with incremental costs, we must begin by properly stating the clinical alternatives to be considered. Suppose a health authority is considering a proposal from a hospital for the purchase of a new sterilization system that will cost Rs. 500,000. The clinical staff of the hospital has reviewed this system and reasonably expects that the new system will reduce nosocomial surgical infections by 90%, over the current system. So at this point, the ICER for this decision would appear in this manner:

(Cost of new system − cost of current system) / (Infection with the new system − infection with the old system)

As we will discuss in a later section, we would purchase the new system if the ICER met the criteria of our decision rule. Now, suppose after discussion with the clinical and bioengineering staff we realize that we have a third option (the first two being to keep our current system and the second to buy the new one) — to upgrade our current system. This will cost only Rs.100,000 and after some study, we believe it will reduce infections by 75%. In this case our decision is now more complicated. We now array these options in Table 11.1.

Table 11.1: Description of economic evaluation problem

Strategy	Cost	Benefit
Keep current system	Rs 5,000*	0% reduction
Upgrade current system	Rs 100,000	75% reduction
Purchase new system	Rs 500,000	90% reduction

*Annual cost of maintenance for current system

Given that the upgrade is the least expensive option and still results in a benefit, we begin by looking at that option.

(Cost of upgrade – cost of current system)/ (Infections with the new system – infections with the old system)

Eq. 11.3: ICER for upgrade of sterilization system

Now, let us assume that we found that the ICER we estimate in Eq. 11.3 meets our criteria for cost-effectiveness. This would mean that we should now consider the upgrade as our best option. Does this mean that we should no longer consider the purchase of the new system? No, what this means is that comparison of the new system with the option of keeping the current system (the ICER estimated in Eq. 11.2) is no longer relevant. We have established that we can reduce infections by 75% by spending Rs.100,000, what we now need to determine is whether it is worth an additional Rs. 400,000 (i.e., the incremental cost of the new system when compared to the upgrade) to reduce infections by an additional 15 percent (i.e., the incremental reduction found with the new system). Note here that we have defined yet a third ICER — one that describes the incremental cost-effectiveness of the new system compared to the upgrade. If this ICER meets our standard of cost-effectiveness we would then purchase the new system; otherwise, we would do the upgrade and be satisfied with a 75% reduction in infections.

The determination that all possible strategies have been considered in answering an economic evaluation question is very important in reviewing the results of economic evaluation studies. The failure to consider less expensive (yet less effective) alternatives will bias the analyses by overstating the true value of more expensive (yet more effective) alternatives.

2. Were the costs and outcomes properly valued?

Before we conduct economic evaluation, we must first know how to properly define costs and benefits. In economic studies, "cost" is properly defined as "*opportunity cost*", that is, the value that would be gained by the next best use of the resource. For instance, suppose that a hospital is considering starting an outpatient diabetes screening program. In order to do so, they must provide space for a waiting area, counseling and equipment. There are many ways we could recognize this cost in our analysis. We could consider what the hospital would charge as rent to a physician or vendor who would want to use that space. We could also consider the cost to the hospital to build and maintain the space. Both of these would be considered "costs" from a traditional accounting or financial perspective. But what is the purpose of the project? Perhaps it is to add a new source of revenue, or to expand services that are needed in the community, or to support a nearby physician practice. In all cases, we want to take the action that benefits the hospital, or alternatively we want to minimize the harm. In either case, benefit or harm is based upon what we give up to do this project.

Suppose that in putting in our screening clinic we make the admittedly absurd decision to take over the waiting area used by patients of our hospital's busiest surgeon. His patients complain to him, he gets angry and takes his clinic to a competing hospital which is happy to provide him with a luxurious office suite. Are our only costs of doing this project the rent we could charge for the space, or the cost to build and maintain it? No, those costs represent but a fraction of what has been lost when the surgeon left. In this case, our *opportunity* cost is the profit we have lost by losing the surgeon's busy practice. Alternatively, suppose we put the screening program in a long vacant part of our campus. Here again, the cost of doing the project is not properly represented by the rent we would charge (no one was paying rent to us in the first place, so how could we lose it?), nor is it the cost of building and maintaining the space (the space already exists and unless we were going to tear it down, we are still going to maintain it). In this case, our opportunity cost associated with this space is zero, because we are not losing anything by giving it up.

Note that is both cases, the opportunity cost is akin to the incremental cost in Eq. 11.1. This is because in these examples opportunity cost is dependent upon the current use of the space. This will not always be the case, but it does point out that opportunity cost and benefit associated with an intervention will vary with the perspective of the decision maker. The most common perspectives considered are the patient, the provider (physician or health system), payer (insurer or governmental entity), or society as a whole. Examining this list you can see how the differences in perspective can affect the characterization of cost and benefit. The charge associated with a procedure is a cost to the patient or payer, while it is a benefit to the provider. The cost associated with delivering a service is irrelevant to the patient or payer, while it is important to the health system or society. A longer life span is a benefit to the patient and society, while it is an element of cost to the payer. Each of these is a legitimate perspective for certain economic evaluations; however, it is generally recommended that when analyses are conducted to affect national or regional coverage policy *the evaluation be conducted from the societal perspective* to ensure that all costs and benefits are considered regardless of source.[8] It is also important to note that in reading reports of economic analyses, the perspective of the analysis should be clearly stated.[7]

3. Was appropriate allowance made for uncertainties in the analysis?

The models used in conducting economic evaluation studies are typically very complex and incorporate data from a number of different sources. A recent report evaluating the cost-effectiveness of glaucoma prevention used a decision-analytic approach with the decision model including over 80 variables incorporating data drawn from clinical studies, reports in the literature, expert opinion, and unpublished data.[6] The results reported from such models are highly dependent upon the assumptions made concerning the variables included and the quality of evidence provided by data sources. In most statistical applications, assessment of the variability of the model is done using confidence intervals, which report the sampling variability. Such an approach is feasible in economic modeling where the primary source of data is a clinical trial, as this allows for estimation of sampling error[8], and there have been a number of methods developed to report such intervals and ellipses.[8,9]

However, as most economic evaluation studies are conducted using decision analytic models incorporating multiple sources of data, use of confidence intervals is rarely practical. Therefore, the more common approach to characterizing the uncertainty of the result is *sensitivity analyses*. In one-way sensitivity analysis the investigator varies each individual parameter (hence, "one-way"), re-estimating the ICER to determine if the change results in a new estimate that would change the cost-effectiveness decision. The full range of clinically relevant values that a parameter may assume must be considered. For example, in a recent American study of grid-laser photocoagulation (GLP)[10], the investigators varied the parameters across a range of ± 10%. The upper limit of this range for the cost of GLP was $1,152 (versus $1,047 used in the model). The reader may question whether this accurately reflects the potential range of average values for a GLP procedure. If not, it calls into question the generalizability of the findings of this investigation.

It is not uncommon for a modest change in one parameter to "sensitize" the model to a change in another. Thus it is important that two-way sensitivity analysis be conducted, where two parameters are varied across a clinically relevant range simultaneously. An example of this was seen in the previously cited report concerning glaucoma prevention. The investigators found that treatment of ocular hypertensives to gain a 40% reduction in their 2% annual risk of developing glaucoma at a cost of $465/year met common standards of cost-effectiveness. They further reported that this decision was very robust to assumptions concerning the cost of treatment, with treatment being cost-effective at a cost of up to $718. However, if the effectiveness decreased by only 5% (resulting in a 35% reduction in risk), then an increase in the cost of treatment to only $612 (i.e., a 30% increase in medication cost) would result in a change in the cost-effectiveness decision.[6]

It is reasonable to assume that the ICER might be influenced by simultaneous changes in a number of variables in a model. This variability is addressed by use of a relatively recent innovation in economic evaluation called probabilistic sensitivity analysis (also known as Monte Carlo simulation). In this technique, each parameter is characterized by a distribution that reflects all clinically relevant values. The investigator uses a software program to "re-sample" each parameter and re-estimate the ICER several thousand times. The proportion of samples for which the intervention was cost-effective compared to the current method of treatment across a range of cost/QALY thresholds is examined to determine how robust the ICER is to the uncertainty of the parameters in the model.[11] We will present an example of this, and discuss interpretation of results later in this chapter.

4. Are estimates of costs and outcomes related to the baseline risk in the treatment population?

Most economic evaluation studies examine the cost-effectiveness of a program to treat or prevent disease on a population basis. This is done by estimating the cost-effectiveness of a "base case"[8] which might be either representative of a single individual who has the average risk factors of one at risk of disease or progression, or a cohort of individuals whose characteristics are representative of those at risk of disease.[6]

However, when considering treatment of an individual patient, or particular subgroup, base case analyses are limited in generalizability. Therefore, it is often necessary to rely on later analyses that examine cost-effectiveness within subgroups to provide direction concerning treatment of individual patients. Recent examples of these include analysis of age[12], gender[13] and other demographic and clinical factors.[14]

II. What Were The Results?

1. What were the incremental costs and outcomes of each strategy?

As noted earlier, it is necessary in constructing the cost-effectiveness analysis that all clinically relevant strategies be considered. Further, we have shown that the incremental costs and benefits associated with each strategy is what are most important. In presenting results, the investigator should present data from which these costs and benefits can be assessed. An example of this is shown in Table 11.2. The investigators compared four potential treatment strategies for glaucoma prevention: (1) treating no one with ocular hypertension (i.e., initiating treatment of ocular hypertension only after the onset of nerve damage); (2) treatment of people with a 5% annual risk of developing glaucoma (referred to as "POAG" in Table 11.2); (3) treatment of people with a 2% annual risk of developing glaucoma; and (4) treatment of all people with ocular hypertension. In Table 10.2, the total costs and benefits (stated in QALYs, discussed below in section III.1) accruing over the relevant period of the analysis are provided. In this example, since the disease being considered is a chronic, non-fatal disease, the period of analysis to be considered is the lifetime.

The investigators found that those with a 5% risk of developing glaucoma represent approximately 10% of those with ocular hypertension. Those with a 2% risk of developing glaucoma are 1/3 of those with ocular hypertension. Obviously, the "Treat no one" strategy would

Table 11.2: Incremental cost-effectiveness of treatment of ocular hypertension to prevent glaucoma (from Kymes et al[6])

Strategy	Total Cost (in $)	Total Effectiveness (QALYs)	Incremental cost ($)	Incremental Effectiveness (QALYs)	Incremental Cost-Effectiveness ratio (cost $/QALYs)
Treat no one	4,006	13.5370			
Treat > 5% annual risk of developing POAG	4,086	13.5588	80	0.0218	3,670
Treat > 2% annual risk of developing POAG	5,308	13.5876	1,222	0.0288	42,430
Treat all persons with ocular hypertension	11,245	13.5870	5,937	–0.0006	Dominated

involve treatment of 0% of those with ocular hypertension and, the "Treat all" strategy would involve treatment of 100%. Table 11.2 dictates the average cost and benefit for each person treated. The row for "Treat no one" indicates that over an average ocular hypertensive's lifetime, they will accrue a cost of $4,006 for treatment of glaucoma and related visual impairment. The incremental cost is detailed in the fourth and fifth columns. From this, we can see in the "Treat 5%" row that treatment of the 10% of ocular hypertensives with the highest risk of glaucoma will cost an additional $80 per person treated and result in a gain of 0.0218 QALYs (or 7.96 quality adjusted life days). Note that this does not indicate that treatment of the 10% of those with the highest risk costs $80 over their lifetime. This is the average across all those at risk, including those not treated. It also includes both the cost of treatment and the savings due to disease prevented.

The "Treat 2%" row details the costs and benefits associated with treatment of the additional 23% of those not treated under the "Treat 5%" strategy. The "Treat all" row details the incremental cost and benefit of treatment of the 67% of ocular hypertensives not treated under the "Treat 2%" strategy. Note that under the ICER column the term "dominated" appears in the "Treat all" row. For this strategy the costs increase, while the benefit decreases. Therefore, in the parlance of economic evaluation, the "Treat all" strategy is said to be dominated by the "Treat ≥ 2%" strategy, as the latter costs less and is more effective than the "Treat all" strategy (The reason for this is a suspected link between treatment of ocular hypertension and an acceleration of cataract development. Therefore, the 67% of those with the lowest risk of glaucoma are at greater risk of developing a cataract than of suffering severe impairment due to glaucoma).

2. How does allowance for uncertainty change the results?

It was not uncommon to report the results of an economic analysis without presenting the associated sensitivity analyses till the recent realization that doing so represents a significant deficiency in the presentation. Characterizing the uncertainty of the result is essential to informing clinicians and policy makers of the practical weight to give the results of the analysis.

Table 11.3: Results of one way sensitivity analyses in evaluation of the treatment of ocular hypertension to prevent glaucoma (adapted from Kymes 2006[6])

Variable	Value in Base Case	Value That Threshold for Treatment Changes from Treat ≥ 2% to Treat ≥ 5%
Incidence of POAG without treatment (all people with ocular hypertension)	2.2%	1.496%
Reduction in risk due to medical treatment	53%	30%
Annual probability of progression of a POAG stage	5.0%	0.5%
Cost of one medication	$465/year	$718
Increased annual risk of cataract surgery due to treatment (additive)	0.33%	2.8%

In Table 11.3, we provide the results of the sensitivity analysis that accompanied the report discussed in Table 11.2. The investigators have identified here those variables which, when altered within a clinically relevant range, change the cost-effectiveness decision (in this application, changing the treatment threshold from those with a 2% annual risk of developing glaucoma, to those with a 5% risk), providing both the value of the variable used in the base case model, and that at which the cost-effectiveness decision would be changed. So,

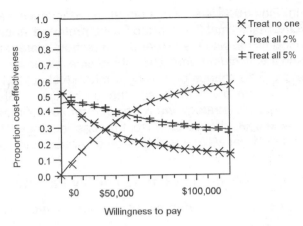

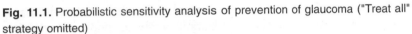

Fig. 11.1. Probabilistic sensitivity analysis of prevention of glaucoma ("Treat all" strategy omitted)

for example, the incidence of glaucoma (i.e., POAG) used in the model was 2.2% (the estimate taken from a large clinical trial[15]). The investigators found that if the mean incidence were to be as low as 1.496%, then a much more conservative treatment threshold (i.e., 5%) would be used rather than what they had initially recommended (i.e., 2%). They went on to explain, using epidemiological evidence, that it was unlikely that the true mean incidence in the sample modeled would be lower than 1.5%, justifying their reliance on the larger estimate and policy recommendation.

The results of probabilistic sensitivity analyses (PSA) are best presented using net-benefit acceptability curves.[11] Curves for the study detailed thus far[6] are presented in Fig. 11.1. The acceptability curve is analogous to confidence intervals more typically seen in association with statistical estimates in that they are a graphic representation of the uncertainty associated with the estimate of cost-effectiveness.

In the PSA process, each parameter is characterized by a distribution, a value is then drawn from that distribution and the ICER re-estimated. This process is repeated a number of times (50,000 in this example) providing a distribution of possible ICERS. The acceptability curve represents the portion of time that the strategy of interest is the "most cost effective" at a certain willingness to pay (as determined by net health benefits[16]; "willingness to pay" is discussed in the next section). In Fig. 10.1, we see that at a willingness to pay of $100,000/QALY the "Treat 2%" strategy is the preferred strategy more than 50% of the time, with the "Treat 5%" threshold preferred 30% of the time, and the "Treat no one" 20% of the time. While it may seem that we have a 50% chance of making a mistake should we choose the "Treat 2%" threshold, what are the alternatives? Should we choose the "Treat 5%" strategy, we will be in error 70% of the time and 80% of the time if we choose the "Treat no one" strategy. Therefore, in this case, the "Treat 2%" threshold seems our best alternative.

III. Will The Results Help in Caring For My Patients?

1.   Are the treatment benefits worth the harms and costs?

There are three methods of economic evaluation commonly used: cost-minimization analysis; cost-benefit analysis; and cost-effectiveness analysis[17] (Fig. 11.2). There is a fourth, cost-utility analysis often cited by authors (and used in our primary example thus far)[3]; however, as we will see, this might be better considered a particularly useful variation of cost-effectiveness analysis. What distinguishes the three methods is the way in which benefit (effectiveness) is measured, and the manner in which the decision rule associated with the ICER is applied.

Where a cost-minimization approach is used, it is assumed that there is no difference in effectiveness between the current standard of practice and the proposed intervention. Therefore, the denominator of

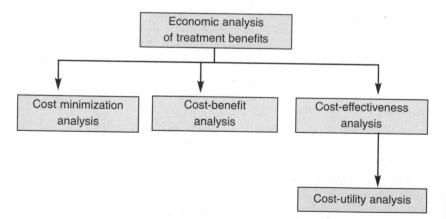

Fig. 11.2. Methods of economic analysis of treatment benefits

the ICER (see Eq. 11.1) is undefined and only the numerator is relevant. The decision rule is that the program with the lowest cost is adopted. This is the method typically used to evaluate a given medication made by different manufacturers, or to compare medication within class. However, it is difficult to be certain that all programs (even generic pharmaceuticals) have completely equal effectiveness. Therefore, most investigators do not consider cost minimization studies optimal for setting health policy.[18]

In cost-benefit analysis, effectiveness of the intervention is characterized in monetary terms, such as the savings due to cost of care avoided, avoidance of lost wages, improved investment due to lower tax burden, etc. If the ICER is greater than 1 (or alternatively applying some algebra to Eq. 11.1: Incremental Benefit of the Intervention − Incremental Cost of the Intervention > 0), then the new health program would be adopted as it provides positive net benefit. Characterizing effectiveness in this manner allows the investigator greater flexibility in comparing health programs, but it has the important limitation that only benefits that can be monetized are considered. For instance, what is the value to be placed on a grandparent with macular degeneration being able to see his/her grandchild? Or, what is the monetary value of being able to read a contract, prescription label, newspaper, or a computer screen? Even if one were able to develop a method to monetize such contributions, it is impossible to argue that such an estimate would be exhaustive. Indeed, because so many benefits of a health intervention are unquantifiable, cost-benefit analysis has limited application where the perspective of analysis is the society or the patient.[8] However, it is very valuable for providers of care and health authorities who must focus their effort on ensuring an operating margin that will provide for the long-term viability of the health program and organization at large.

In cost-effectiveness analysis, the effectiveness of the intervention is characterized in "natural" (i.e., non-monetary) units. These might be "years of life saved", "cases of blindness avoided", "years of disability avoided", etc. While cost-effectiveness analysis allows consideration of both monetary and non-monetary benefits of a health program, interpretation of the results is not as straightforward as seen in cost-minimization and cost-benefit analyses. In cost-effectiveness analyses, the ICER informs the decision maker of the cost to "purchase" each incremental natural unit gained (or avoided, where the outcome is negative). Determining cost-effectiveness then requires that a decision-maker know what is the value of the natural unit (i.e., year of life, case of blindness, disability).

A recent report by Lairson and colleagues reported that prophylactic use of acyclovir to prevent recurrence of ocular herpes simplex (HSV) costs $8,532 per recurrence prevented.[19] The results beg the question: what is the value of preventing recurrence of ocular herpes? This of course depends on the perspective, and in the case of this report the perspective was that of society as a whole. Interestingly, both the investigators and an accompanying editorial[20] suggest that it is less than $8,532, but could provide no evidence, empirical or otherwise, to support this argument.

One way to address this begins by assuming that "society" as a decision maker can be represented by an "average" person. In this case, assume that an average person exists, who has not yet contracted HSV, but properly understands her risk of doing so, as well as the risk of recurrence. She also has good understanding of what impairment and pain HSV may cause and its impact on her quality of life. She (not her insurer, government, or other third-party payer) will fully bear the cost of treatment if she contracts HSV. Now, as someone who has never had the disease, we ask her to decide whether it would be "worth it" to pay $8,532 to prevent recurrence of HSV (if she were to contract the disease). If she says yes, it would be cost-effective for society to implement this program, if she says "No", it would not be.

Answering this question is the purpose of cost-utility analysis. In cost-utility analysis, the "natural unit" considered is the "quality adjusted life year" (QALY). The QALY is a measure of benefit that considers not only prevention of disease, but the impact of the disease on quality of life by weighing the person's expected lifespan by a measure of quality of life referred to as the *utility*. This is a measure of a person's perception of quality of life that is generally bounded by 0 and 1, with zero representing death and one, perfect health.[21] There are three primary methods for measuring utility: the visual analog scale (VAS), the standard gamble (SG), and the time trade-off (TTO). In the VAS, the person is asked to rate their perception of health state on a line with one end being death and the other perfect health.[3] In the latter two methods the person is asked to consider what he/she would "trade" to gain perfect health (in SG, the risk of immediate death, in TTO a portion of the person's remaining life span).[22] The latter two methods are considered to be the most consistent with economic theory.[23]

Cost-utility analysis is particularly well suited to evaluation of chronic, disabling diseases that have significant impact on quality of life. It allows the length of time spent living with the disease (or without, in the case of prevention) as well as its impact on quality of life to be considered. In cost-utility analysis, the ICER provides an estimate of the cost of "purchasing" an additional year of "perfect" health. For instance, in the cost-utility analysis described thus far in this chapter the investigators found that at a treatment threshold of $\geq$ 2%, treatment of people with ocular hypertension to prevent glaucoma had an ICER of $42,430 (see Table 10.2) This implies that employing such a treatment strategy would require the expenditure of over $42,430 for each quality adjusted life year (QALY) gained.[6]

This approach requires the decision makers to consider how much "society" is willing to "spend" for a year of perfect health (i.e., one QALY). Unfortunately, there is little consensus on this question among policy makers. For over 20 years, the informal standard in the West was considered to be[24] $50,000, but some authors have provided compelling evidence that the true value most industrialized nations place on the QALY is[25] over $200,000. However, while there is limited empirical evidence to support such claims, most investigators generally believe[26] that the appropriate standard in the industrialized world lies between $50,000 and100,000. This question has not been addressed in any detail by investigators from the Third World, but it would be reasonable to suppose that such societies may place a lower value on a QALY given the lower cost of living and differing social perspectives.

2. Could my patients expect similar health outcomes?

The issue of whether the results reported from an economic evaluation will be similar to those seen in a different setting is of course a question of generalizability. What will determine this are the factors: (1) are the characteristics seen in the patients similar to those whose characteristics are modeled in the economic evaluation?; and (2) were the clinical procedures employed in the intervention modeled similar to those which would be used in the practice setting?[7]

However, it is not always the case that significant deviations in patient characteristics or clinical procedures will result in a substantially different cost-effectiveness decision. Sensitivity analysis will give important direction on this. In the study of glaucoma prevention[6], Kymes and colleagues modeled a hypothetical cohort representative of the age distribution of people with ocular hypertension. In their report, they indicated that they tested the influence of age distribution on the cost-effectiveness decision, and found that the result was not sensitive to changes in this risk factor. Therefore, if consideration were being made to apply this clinical policy in a community that is older (or younger) than those modeled, that fact should not influence the decision of the policy maker. On the other hand, as reported in Table 11.3, the overall risk of glaucoma in the cohort modeled was 2.2%/year. Therefore, if clinical characteristics of the community are such that the risk of glaucoma is lower than average, the policy maker may reconsider whether the results of this study are applicable in her/his community. Similarly, we also see in Table 11.3 important factors related to clinical practice. As is seen in most modeling exercises, Kymes et al. based their model upon clinical practice guidelines from the American Academy of Ophthalmology. Therefore, in the model, clinical follow-up and treatment decisions would be similar to those defined in the guideline. Such decisions may affect several factors seen in Table 11.3, particularly the risk of progression, incidence of cataract surgery, and reduction in risk (which might be related to patient compliance). If local practice deviates from those modeled in the guideline and such deviations affect these factors, the decision maker needs to carefully evaluate whether similar cost-effectiveness outcomes will be seen.

3.   Could I expect similar costs?

Costs of interventions will always be very specific to the jurisdiction in which the evaluation is conducted. It is due to this that while one can rely on sensitivity analyses to evaluate the generalizability of results as they relate to clinical characteristics or practice, it is more difficult to make such evaluations relating to cost.

In the example presented in Tables 11.2 and 11.3, the cost of medication is presented as an influential factor in the cost-effectiveness decision. It is doubtful whether ocular anti-hypertensive medication will be priced in a similar manner in a developing nation (or even another industrialized nation) as it will be in the United States (where this evaluation was conducted); therefore, one would be cautious about making generalizations concerning this study across countries. However, it is even more important to realize that it is not simply the level of cost of a single input (or several inputs) that influences the ICER, but the overall relationship of the costs to each other.[7] Therefore, if the cost of medication in India is 1/3 the cost in the United States (after adjustment for currency), the cost-effectiveness decision would remain unchanged so long as all the costs incorporated in the model were similarly lower. However, if the relationship between the costs differs significantly (i.e., the cost of medication in India is 1/3 of that seen in the U.S., but the cost of treating glaucoma is 1/10th of that seen in the U. S.), the potential for bias in the result would be substantial due to the complex relationship of variables in the economic model. Therefore, under these conditions it would be necessary to conduct an analysis specific to the new jurisdiction. Economic evaluation forms a critical element in the appraisal of the value and significance of healthcare interventions when viewed from a variety of important perspectives – that of a patient, payer, provider or society. Established principles provide explicit guidance in the appropriate methodology best suited to provide care and conduct tests. A working knowledge of these guidelines is enormously useful for any clinician, administrator or health researcher.

References

1. Anderson GF, et al. It's the prices stupid: why the United States is so different from other countries. *Health Affairs.* 2003; 22(3): 89-105.

2. Drummond MF, et al. *Methods for the Economic Evaluation of Health Care Programmes.* 3rd ed. Oxford: Oxford University Press; 2005.

3. Frick KD, et al. Estimating the burden and economic impact of trachomatous visual loss. *Ophthalmic Epidemiology.* 2003; 10(2): 121-32.

4. Frick KD, Colchero MA, Dean D. Modeling the economic net benefit of a potential vaccination program against ocular infection with Chlamydia trachomatis.[see comment]. *Vaccine.* 2004; 22(5-6): 689-96.

5. Frick KD, Hanson CL, Jacobson GA. Global burden of trachoma and economics of the disease. American Journal of Tropical Medicine & Hygiene. 2003; 69(5 Suppl): 1-10.

6. Kymes SM, et al. Management of ocular hypertension: a cost-effectiveness approach from the ocular hypertension treatment study. *American Journal of Ophthalmology.* 2006; 141(6): 997-1008.

7. O'Brien B, et al. Users' Guides to the Medical Literature: XIII. How to use an article on economic analysis of clinical practice B. what are the results and will they help me in caring for my patients? *JAMA.* 1997; 277(22): 1802-6.

8. Gold MR, et al. *Cost-Effectiveness in Health and Medicine.* 1st ed. ed. Gold MR. New York: Oxford University Press; 1996.

9. Polsky D, et al. Confidence intervals for cost-effectiveness ratios: a comparison of four methods. *Health Economics,* 1997; 6: 243-52.

10. Sharma S, et al. The cost-effectiveness of grid laser photocoagulation for the treatment of diabetic macular edema: results of a patient-based cost-utility analysis. *Current Opinion in Ophthalmology.* 2000; 11(3): 175-9.

11. Fenwick E, Claxton K, Sculpher M. Representing uncertainty: the role of cost-effectiveness acceptability curves. *Health Economics.* 2001; 10: 779-87.

12. Russell LB, Sisk JE. Modeling age differences in cost-effectiveness analysis. a review of the literature. *International Journal of Technology Assessment in Health Care*, 2000; 16(4): 1158-67.
13. Kanis JA, et al. Cost-effectiveness of preventing hip fracture in the general female population. *Osteoporosis International*. 2001; 12(5): 356-61.
14. Nixon RM, Thompson SG, Methods for incorporating covariate adjustment, subgroup analysis and between-centre differences into cost-effectiveness evaluations. *Health Economics*. 2005;14(12): 1217-29.
15. Kass MA, et al. The ocular hypertension treatment study: a randomized trial determines that topical hypotensive medication delays or prevents the onset of primary open-angle glaucoma. *Archives of Ophthalmology*. 2002; 120: 701-13.
16. Stinnett AA, Mullahy J. Net health benefits: a new framework for the analysis of uncertainty in cost-effectiveness analysis. *Medical Decision Making*, 1998; 18(2 (Supplement)): S68-S80.
17. Meltzer MI. Introduction to health economics for physicians.[see comment]. *Lancet*. 2001; 358(9286): 993-8.
18. Briggs AH, O'Brien BJ. The death of cost-minimization analysis. *Health Economics Letters*, 2000; 4(4): 3-10.
19. Lairson DR, et al. Prevention of herpes simplex virus eye disease: a cost-effectiveness analysis.[see comment]. Archives of Ophthalmology. 2003; 121(1): 108-12.
20. Lee P, Zhang P. Economic analysis in eye disease. *Archives of Ophthalmology*. 2003; 121(1): 115-16.
21. Torrance GW, Feeny DH. Utilities and quality adjusted life years. *International Journal of Technology Assessment in Health Care*. 1989; 5: 559-75.
22. Torrance GW. Social preferences for health states: an empirical evaluation of three measurement techniques. *Social Science and Medicine*. 1976; 10: 129-136.
23. Kymes SM, Frick KD. Value based medicine.[comment]. *British Journal of Ophthalmology*. 2005; 89(5): 643-4; author reply, 644.
24. Hirth RA, et al. Willingness to pay for a quality-adjusted life year: in search of a standard. *Medical Decision Making*. 2000; 20(3): 332-42.
25. Ubel PA, et al. What is the price of life and why doesn't it increase with the rate of inflation? *Archives of Internal Medicine*. 2003; 163: 1637-41.
26. Gillick MR. Medicare coverage for technological innovations - time for new criteria? *New England Journal of Medicine*. 2004; 350(21): 2199-2203.
27. Drummond MF, Richardson WS, O'Brien BJ, Levine M, Heyland D. Users' Guides to the Medical Literature. XIII. How to use an article on economic analysis of clinical practice. A. Are the results of the study valid? *JAMA*, 1997; 277(19):1552-7.

12

Translating EBM into Practice

Ajit N. Babu

- Roadblocks in the Way of EBM
- Insufficient Time
- Lack of Access to Evidence
- Contradictory Evidence for Many Clinical Issues
- Skepticism and Doubt about EBM from Peers or Superiors
- Conclusion

Roadblocks in the Way of EBM

We have discussed at length some of the theory behind EBM and the projected benefits of using it in clinical practice. All would agree though that there can be a world of difference between theory and practice. EBM can be difficult to implement in real-world situations for a variety of reasons (Fig. 12.1), like:

- Insufficient time
- Lack of access to evidence
- Contradictory evidence for many clinical issues
- Skepticism and doubt about EBM from peers or superiors

Under these problematic circumstances, it is important to evolve practical methods of using EBM when appropriate. We shall consider each of the above factors in detail.

Insufficient Time

The biggest constraint in many clinical settings is a lack of time. Particularly, when patient volumes are high, it may simply not be practical to search for evidence, critically appraise it and take a decision. What can a clinician do then to apply EBM in day-to-day practice? It requires

Insufficient time

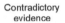

Skepticism of
superiors

Lack of access
to evidence

Contradictory
evidence

Fig. 12.1. Roadblocks in the way of EBM practice

common sense thinking and a balanced approach. Key elements
include the following:

- Point of care information
- Collected resources
- Selective review

Point of care information

The most useful evidence is that which is available at the time and
place wherein its application is decisive and required – this is known
as the **point of care**. For it to be feasible, the best evidence source
would be electronic media – either the Internet, or programs loaded
on to a computer, especially one which also runs an electronic medical record (EMR) that could either have seamless access to such
data which reside outside the EMR, or have a specific module as part
of the EMR that meets this function. In the absence of electronic
media, even printed matter such as textbooks, journals, practice
guidelines and so on are also sources for evidence, though as we
have discussed in earlier chapters, textbooks may not be ideal for getting access to the latest information. They are certainly useful, however, for giving a multifaceted overview of a topic, and reviewing generally accepted and established therapies.

Collected resources

A familiar example is the medical library where there is a large collection of medical knowledge under one roof. Increasingly, even in Third World settings, libraries encompass not just the traditional assemblage of textbooks and journals, but also electronic resources like on-line subscription to texts and journals, specially designed online composite resources, and multimedia programs that deal with specific medical topics. Medical knowledge resources like the library or online repositories (a "digital library") are commonly being viewed as a form of medical information just like patient records, and these areas are frequently coming under a common administrative umbrella. Digital libraries have the great advantage of being accessible from any designated computer within the institutional network and often even from the outside over the Internet. This is an excellent way of improving access to evidence, since multiple users can potentially access a given resource simultaneously – something that is not possible with a paper resource that has only a single copy. More about online resources is covered in Chapter 6.

Selective review

This is essentially the application of common sense to our pursuit of EBM. From a thoughtful analysis of our own practice patterns, it is possible to identify the common clinical conditions that we encounter on a regular basis. For example, an internist may regularly see hypertension, diabetes mellitus, coronary artery disease, febrile illnesses and so on. It would be eminently feasible to focus one's reading on disorders like this while time and resources are available to update and enhance one's own knowledge base. It will then become much easier to practice EBM at the point of care since you will not have to expend time and effort in actually trying to find evidence in the clinic while the patient is sitting in front of you. Inpatient practice lends itself to EBM application more easily since there is usually time to review evidence, while the patient remains in the hospital. However, even under this circumstance, it is prudent to have reviewed common clinical problems seen in the wards to optimize the efficiency of the care provided.

Lack of Access to Evidence

The problem of lack of access to evidence can be due to two main reasons – either the evidence exists but is not accessible due to constraints of logistics, or the evidence does not exist at all. Since there is not much that can be done to resolve the latter issue at the level of the individual practitioner, let us concentrate on the former.

Evidence can be presented in two primary formats: paper and electronic. Between the two, the latter medium is far more versatile and useful given the diversity of information it can make available to the user, with the provision for constant updating and revision. A paper resource like a textbook may be cheaper and convenient in that it is accessible even in settings where there is no power and retrieving information may be as simple as looking up in the index. There are also two types of evidence sources – primary evidence, where the actual evidence is directly presented to the reader, and secondary evidence, where available evidence has been reviewed and collated into a comprehensive document or summary with the advantage of saving time for the reader and adding an expert perspective. It is essential in this day and age to have computer access, and it can no longer be regarded as a luxury. The rest of the discussion will focus on electronic resources. As noted in Chapter 6, there are a variety of free online resources out of which the most valuable may well be *PubMed* provided by courtesy of the National Library of Medicine, Bethesda, MD, USA. It allows one to retrieve not only citations of journal articles with abstracts from MEDLINE, but also has direct links to available free full-text resources from the citation page. *PubMed Central* is a related resource that has free full-text archives from hundreds of journals, including some prestigious ones like *BMJ*. A useful free resource of collected information that has some EBM elements is eMedicine. A number of paid sources are also popular internationally, perhaps the leading provider being *Up To Date,* which is a subscription service that is updated three times a year, and includes web access as well as content storable on a PC and a PDA (Personal Digital Assistant). It is unfortunately rather expensive and may be beyond the reach of those without adequate financial resources to draw upon. To learn more about the actual process of EBM, the best online resources are the *JAMA* Users' Guides to the Medical Literature (by free subscription) and the Evidence-based Practice site hosted by the Centre for Health Evidence. Website addresses to all of these resources are given at the end of the chapter.

Contradictory Evidence for Many Clinical Issues

It is sad but true that there is often little agreement on important clinical issues from either the perspective of evidence or among experts.

When faced with this difficult situation, the practitioner would be well advised to go with the best-designed studies that have the greatest generalizability to their particular practice environment. There are times when even getting to this point in the decision-making process is an insurmountable challenge. It is in these difficult situations that clinical judgment has to weigh in and support a definite course of action. Though the ambiguity inherent in such an approach can be disheartening, it is worth considering the bright side – these complexities make it exceedingly unlikely that an omnipotent computer will replace the clinician anytime in the near future!

Skepticism and Doubt about EBM from Peers or Superiors

There are many who either have no knowledge of EBM and its foundations, or who regard it as a dubious enterprise, even when they might acknowledge the value of a scientific method applied to medical practice. Many of the great innovations in history ranging from the telephone to electricity were met with initial ridicule and pessimism. Compared to these wonderful discoveries, EBM is rather tame in its change from tradition! It is in fact built on many well-established principles of clinical epidemiology that originated decades ago – the key difference is the way in which it has been packaged and applied in a user-friendly fashion. The best way to win over a skeptic is to show them how EBM can operate in real life to answer clinical questions and suggest the most rational approach to clinical care. A nice opportunity in academic settings where there is a "journal club" is to use EBM techniques for the critical appraisal part. The more structured and knowledgeable review that becomes possible may be an eye-opener to some. In fairness, it must also be said that the budding EBM practitioner has to recognize that there may be many situations in which EBM cannot generate a clear answer. Like any technique, EBM works in certain settings but not in others and one should not blindly try to apply it in a reflexive fashion. Given the variations in resources like computer access, online material, and time available in a given clinical environment, there is no doubt that there will be places and practices where EBM is logistically very difficult to follow, even if it would have been otherwise appropriate. It is the wise practitioner who can recognize his/her practice milieu and fashion clinical work in a manner that will work best within his/her resources and constraints.

Conclusion

EBM promises advancements in our approach to patient care. There are, however, a number of practical difficulties in implementing EBM in real-world settings. Lack of time, insufficient access to evidence, contradictory findings from available evidence and skepticism from seniors or peers can all contribute to the challenge. Availability of point of care information, collected resources (particularly online) and a selective approach to reviewing evidence related to common clinical conditions are helpful in making EBM work for you, at least most of the time. EBM evokes a range of responses – from the sarcastic scoffers who jeer at the process to the fanatical foot soldiers of the EBM movement who stalk their peers with glazed eyes looking to add another EBM scalp to their swelling kitty. The real truth, as always, lies somewhere between these extremes – and the reader will no doubt find his or her own level of comfort over time. Till then – drive carefully!

Table 12.1: What can you actually do?

1. Read about your patients.
2. Identify commonly encountered clinical problems - review and revise knowledge.
3. Try to get the "best available" evidence.
4. Improve access to evidence.
5. Think about what you are doing and why.
6. Don't forget the patient while pursuing the evidence...

Recommended Resources

1. Clinicians for the Restoration of Autonomous Practice Writing Group. EBM: unmasking the ugly truth. *BMJ*. 2002; 325:1496-1498.
2. Evidence-Based Medicine Working Group. Evidence-based medicine: a new approach to teaching the practice of medicine. *JAMA*. 1992; 268:2420-2425.
3. Fletcher RH, Fletcher SW, Wagner EH. *Clinical Epidemiology: The Essentials*. 3rd ed. Baltimore: Williams & Wilkins; 1996.
4. Guyatt GH, Rennie D. Users' guides to the medical literature. *JAMA*. 1993; 270:2096-2097.
5. Oxman AD, Sackett DL, Guyatt GH. For the Evidence-Based Medicine Working Group. Users' guides to the medical literature, I: how to get started. *JAMA*. 1993; 270:2093-2095.

6. Sackett DL, Haynes RB, Guyatt GH, Tugwell P. *Clinical Epidemiology: A Basic Science for Clinical Medicine.* 2nd ed. Boston, Mass: Little Brown & Co Inc; 1991:145-148.
7. Sackett DL, Straus SE, Richardson WS, et al. *Evidence-Based Medicine: How to Practice and Teach EBM.* Toronto, Ontario: Churchill Livingstone; 1998.
8. Centre for Health Evidence User's Guide to Evidence-based Practice at: http://www.cche.net/usersguides/main.asp
9. eMedicine at: http://www.emedicine.com/
10. JAMA Users' Guides to the Medical Literature at: http://ugi.usersguides. org/usersguides/hg/hh_start.asp
11. PubMed at: http://www.ncbi.nlm.nih.gov/entrez/query.fcgi?db=PubMed
12. PubMed Central at: http://www.pubmedcentral.nih.gov/
13. UpToDate at: http://www.uptodate.com/

13

Evidence–based Medicine and Medical Informatics: The Role of Clinical Decision Support Systems (CDSS)

Suptendra Nath Sarbadhikari

■ Relationship between
Evidence-based Medicine
and Medical Informatics

  ● How can MI principles
  and techniques help in
  better EBM practice
  with special reference
  to CDSS?

■ Practical Examples

■ Conclusions and Future
Directions

Relationship between Evidence-based Medicine and Medical Informatics

EBM (Evidence–based Medicine) is the conscientious, explicit and judicious use of current best evidence for making decisions about care of individual patient, in a scientific and systematic manner[1]. Its primary areas of emphasis (Fig. 13.1) lie in (a) decisions in clinical medicine, (b) therapeutic evaluations, (c) preventive strategies and screening, (d) healthcare policies, (e) health economics and (f) research and innovations. An essential adjunct to the practice of evidence-based medicine (EBM) is medical informatics (MI) that focuses on creating tools to access and apply the best evidence for making decisions about patient care[1].

Before practicing EBM, practitioners must be familiar with medical journals, literature databases, medical textbooks, practice guidelines, and the growing number of other dedicat-

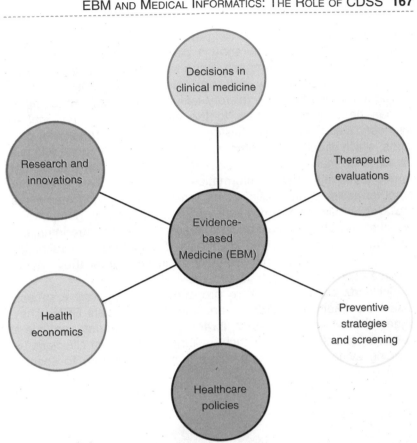

Fig. 13.1. Areas of emphasis of evidence-based medicine (EBM)

ed evidence-based resources, like the Cochrane Database of Systematic Reviews and Clinical Evidence[2]. Similarly, for practicing medical informatics properly, it is essential to have an understanding of EBM, including the ability to phrase an answerable question, locate and retrieve the best evidence, and critically appraise and apply it[3,4]. Reaching a confident diagnosis is never an easy job for a clinician, and frequently the final diagnosis can be in doubt till time or repeated investigation reveals the answer. Often, a simple diagnostic procedure or test is overlooked initially and the disease eludes diagnosis. Clinical reasoning and decision-making are phased[5-7]. Initially, there is a clinical evaluation, followed by indicated laboratory investigations. Integration of clinical findings and test results follow. After that, com-

parative benefits and risks are weighed among the alternative courses of actions. Finally, a therapeutic plan is developed taking into
account the patient's preferences, along with ethical and other considerations like cost of therapy, and compliance expectations.

Right from the first step (history taking) to the final one, computers can be of immense help to the clinician. *CDSS (Clinical or
Diagnostic Decision Support Systems* [7] are interactive computer programs, which directly assist physicians and other health professionals
with decision-making tasks. They reflect a practical application that
marries EBM with medical informatics (Fig. 13.2). Nevertheless, for
computer-assisted diagnostic systems, a human clinician ("man in the
loop" for Intelligence Amplification) is an essential component.
Moreover, the clinician must understand completely the strengths and
limitations of computer-aided diagnosis. Computerized diagnostics
and clinical acumen are not mutually exclusive; rather they should
reinforce each other for optimal results.

Schwartz and Millam[8] have proposed an interesting approach
outside the traditional CDSS where informatics assists EBM. They
suggest that a web-based EBM library consult model may provide a
useful way for informaticians such as librarians to assist clinicians by
providing evidence-based responses from the literature to specific
clinical queries.

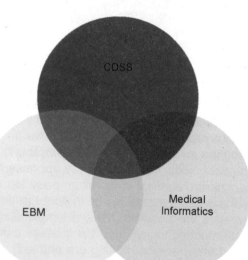

Fig. 13.2. CDSS depends on a combination of EBM with medical informatics.

How can MI Principles and Techniques Help in Better EBM Practice with Special Reference to CDSS?

CDSS offer a powerful MI tool that can be usefully applied to EBM practice. Other applications of informatics that are ubiquitous in clinical practice nowadays are the use of resources like the Internet and *PubMed* to look up published medical information, journals and even patient-centered informational sites or support groups. Finally, knowledge bases such as online versions of popular textbooks and medical databases are growing exponentially in their use, especially by younger clinicians who are increasingly comfortable with computing and applied informatics as a part of their daily practice. This chapter will look at the interface of EBM and CDSS in more detail, as other EBM related applications of informatics are dealt with in more detail in Chapter 5.

At every step of the medical diagnostic process, there are scopes for *ambiguities* in inputs such as: (a) *history* (patient's description of the diseased condition – a relative degree of threshold for suffering, or quality of expression of complaints), (b) *physical examination* (especially in cases of uncooperative or less intelligent patients), and (c) *laboratory tests* (faulty methods or equipment). Moreover, in *treatment*, there are chances of: (a) drug reactions and specific allergies, and (b) patients non-compliance of the therapy due to cost or time or adverse reactions. All these have to be encoded properly to form a working CDSS. The basic components of a CDSS are: (a) knowledge base and (b) inference mechanism. The advantages are that they are prompt, logical, definitive, prone to less chance of errors, purveying stepwise checklists, likely to avoid unnecessary expensive tests, and remotely networkable. The inherent limitations to any CDSS are that (a) final solution may be unknown and (b) the "man in the loop" is essential.

The early models for building a Knowledge Base and utilizing it for decision-making were:

a. Logical/deductive: branching logic (e.g., ID3 or iterative dichotomizer 3), e.g., MYCIN, NEOMYCIN[9]]

b. Probabilistic: Bayesian[10], e.g., de Dombal and

c. Hybrid: heuristic reasoning, e.g., QMR, DXplain, ILIAD

QMR (Quick Medical Reference) is a multifaceted computer program for internal medicine. It can generate a differential diagnosis from clinical information entered into its program, offer information on over 600 diseases, describe associated disorders and complications of diseases, offer strategies to confirm or exclude disorders, and provide simulated cases for educational purposes[11]. Dxplain has similar capabilities, and was developed by the computer science laboratory at the Massachusetts General Hospital, Boston.

Computer-based diagnostic systems are available commercially, but there has been limited evaluation of their performance. Berner et al[12] had assessed the diagnostic capabilities of four internal medicine diagnostic systems: *Dxplain, Iliad, Meditel,* and QMR. Ten expert clinicians created a set of 105 diagnostically challenging clinical case summaries involving actual patients. Clinical data were entered into each program with the vocabulary provided by the program's developer. Each of the systems produced a ranked list of possible diagnoses for each patient, as did the group of experts. No single computer program outscored the others on all performance measures. Among all cases and all programs, the proportion of correct diagnoses ranged from 0.52 to 0.71, and the mean proportion of relevant diagnoses ranged from 0.19 to 0.37. On average, less than half the diagnoses on the experts' original list of reasonable diagnoses were suggested by any of the programs. However, each program suggested an average of approximately two additional diagnoses per case that the experts found relevant but had not originally considered. These results reflect the strengths and limitations of the evaluated programs and can be reasonably extrapolated to the likely performance of other similarly designed CDSS. To gain the maximal benefit from such programs, physicians would need to use their clinical discrimination and common sense to weed out the relevant suggestions from the unlikely ones.

Presently the active assistant or clinical event monitor, e.g., HELP, CPMC models are preferred. Integrated CDSS combines CBR (case based reasoning), ANN (artificial neural networks), Bayesian, Procedural, and Production Rule methods in various proportions, in accordance with the need[7].

In another study, Bergman and Fors[13] have investigated how different preferences of Learning Styles (LS) of psychiatrists might affect acceptance, use and perceived usefulness of a CDSS for diagnostics in psychiatry. The LS preferences of the 49 physicians turned out as follows: 37% were Assimilating, 31% Converging, 27% Accommodating and 6% Diverging. The CDSS under study seemed to favor psychiatrists with abstract conceptualization information perceiving mode (Assimilating and Converging learning styles). A correlation between learning styles preferences and computer skill was found. Positive attitude to computer-aided diagnostics and learning styles preferences was also found to correlate. Using the CDSS, the specialists produced only 1 correct diagnosis and the non-specialists 2 correct diagnoses (median values) as compared to the three predetermined correct diagnoses of the actual case. Only 10% had all three diagnoses correct, 41 % two correct, 47 % one correct and 2 % had no correct diagnoses at all. These findings indicate that the use of CDSS does not guarantee correct diagnosis and that LS might influence the results.

Tan et al[14] performed a Cochrane Review and concluded that there are very limited data from randomized trials on which to assess the effects of clinical decision support systems in neonatal care.

Garg et al[15] feel that developers of healthcare software have attributed improvements in patient care to these applications. As with any healthcare intervention, such claims require confirmation in clinical trials. They updated their earlier reviews by searching the MEDLINE, EMBASE, Cochrane Library, Inspec, and ISI databases and consulting reference lists through September 2004. Authors of 64 primary studies confirmed data or provided additional information. They included randomized and nonrandomized controlled trials that evaluated the effect of a CDSS compared with care provided without a CDSS on practitioner performance or patient outcomes. Teams of 2 reviewers independently abstracted data on methods, setting, CDSS and patient characteristics, and outcomes. One hundred studies met their inclusion criteria. The number and methodological quality of studies improved over time. The CDSS improved practitioner performance in 62 (64%) of the 97 studies assessing this outcome, including 4 (40%) of 10 diagnostic systems, 16 (76%) of 21 reminder systems, 23 (62%) of 37 disease management systems, and 19 (66%) of 29 drug-dosing or prescribing systems. Fifty-two trials assessed 1 or more patient outcomes, of which 7 trials (13%) reported improvements. Improved practitioner performance was associated with CDSSs that automatically prompted users compared with requiring users to activate the system (success in 73% of trials vs. 47%; P = .02) and studies in which the authors also developed the CDSS software compared with studies in which the authors were not the developers (74% success vs. 28%; respectively, P = .001). They concluded that many CDSS programs improve practitioner performance. However, our understanding of the true impact of CDSS on patient outcomes remains nebulous at best.

A related term to CDSS the reader may be familiar with is "Expert System". **Expert Systems (ES)** are complex AI (artificial intelligence) programs. The most widely used way of representing domain knowledge in ES is as a set of production rules, which are often coupled with a frame system that defines the objects that occurs in the rules.

Connectionist ES are ANN based ES where the ANN generates inferencing rules, e.g., fuzzy-MLP where linguistic and natural forms of inputs are used. Apart from that, rough set theory may be used for encoding knowledge in the weights better and also GAs (genetic algorithms) may be used to optimize the search for better, faster results.

Sim et al[16] had proposed to capture literature-based and practice-based evidence in machine-interpretable knowledge bases; develop maintainable technical and methodological foundations for computer-based decision support; evaluate the clinical effects and costs of clinical decision support systems and the ways clinical decision support systems affect and are affected by professional and organizational practices; identify and disseminate best practices for work flow-sensitive implementations of clinical decision support systems; and establish public policies that provide incentives for implementing clinical decision support systems to improve healthcare quality. They introduced a new term, "evidence-adaptive CDSS," to distinguish a type of CDSS that has technical and methodological requirements that are not shared by CDSS programs in general. Here, the clinical knowledge base of the CDSS is derived from and continually reflects the most up-to-date evidence from the research literature and practice-based sources. For example, a CDSS for cancer treatment is evidence-adaptive if its knowledge base is based on current evidence and if its recommendations are routinely updated to incorporate new research findings. Conversely, a CDSS that alerts clinicians to a known drug–drug interaction is evidence-based but not evidence-adaptive if its clinical knowledge base is derived from scientific evidence, but no mechanisms are in place to incorporate new research findings.

Haynes[17] provided a "4S" hierarchical structure, with original "studies" at the base, "syntheses" (systematic reviews) of evidence just above the base, "synopses" of studies and syntheses coming next up, and the most evolved evidence based information "systems" at the top. Information seekers should begin looking at the highest-level resource available for the problem that prompted their search. Kunnamo et al[18] have proposed to establish a comprehensive national decision support database and provide it as a free web service for electronic patient record suppliers in Finland. Their comprehensive decision support system aims to cover various elements of clinical decision making both in primary and secondary care. They report that the project has been welcomed by practicing physicians, and it has received national funding. The script descriptions are written in simple English, and the functions of the scripts and the data they require are described in detail. The evidence is stated clearly and quantitatively, and links are made to evidence summaries and guidelines at www.ebm-guidelines.com. Potential harms are described separately, because the ethical requirements of implementing automated decision support are strict. The output (reminders) of the scripts is in Finnish and English languages, and other languages can be easily added. Authoring, programming and testing one script is stated to take a total of one day of the author and programmer's time, if evidence summaries already exist. A common web-based tool for obtaining referee comments was developed for both Current Care national guidelines and for the decision support database. The first scripts were produced about diabetes and cardiovascular risk factors. Calculators such as the SCORE calculator for estimating cardiovascular have been included. The testing of the scripts has started within a diabetes management system that provided diagnoses, medications, laboratory results, blood pressure readings, weight, and height to be processed by the scripts. Qualitative research on the usability and acceptability of the system has been started in the form of focus group meetings, and a randomized intervention study is being planned to assess the impact of the system on health personnel performance and patient outcomes.

Steinberg and Luce[19] show how decision-making is an integral part of successful implementation of EBM. The reasons that real-world decisions regarding healthcare are often so difficult to make are: the potential nature and magnitude of the impact of a healthcare intervention; the best estimate of the probability that those impacts will occur; the uncertainty surrounding that estimate, as reflected in the strength of available evidence regarding safety and efficacy; the uncertainty surrounding that estimate as a result of uncertainty regarding the generalizability of study findings to other patient populations or care settings (efficacy versus effectiveness); the fact that data from studies regarding an intervention's impacts are not always available; the consequences of being wrong from different people's or entities' perspectives; and costs in light of limited resources and potential alternative uses of them.

Practical Examples

Let us discuss the role of processing information (informatics!), before starting the actual search in cyberspace, with a couple of examples.

A 70-year-old man, presenting to the casualty at night, complains of loss of energy, trouble concentrating, decreased appetite, and insomnia. He has lost considerable weight since his last visit and appears disheveled. How would you approach this case?

On reviewing this scenario, you can easily see the age group of the man ("geriatric" or "elderly") and also that he has symptoms suggestive of some form of "depression" (may be primary or secondary which has to be determined later). Here, the best way to find evidence will be to frame a search phrase like "geriatric depression differential diagnosis" and search through popular online resources like Google or eMedicine. On the other hand, if you try to find answers to each of the symptoms randomly in the World Wide Web, you may not get the answer to the question of exactly how to approach such a case – what are the emergency precautions to be taken? If you go through the first 3 or 4 pages retrieved with the above search phrase from popular resources such as Google or eMedicine, you come to know the increased risk of suicide in such a case and exactly what questions should be asked to get a hint about his suicidal ideation and state of mind. Also, the importance of the drug and alcohol history, medication history and family history would become readily apparent.

A person from South Africa appears to be suffering from lethal encephalitis. What could be the causative agents?

In this particular case, the key words are "lethal encephalitis" and "Africa". Therefore, the search phrase should include these terms. Google will return with "West Nile Fever", "Trypanosomiasis" and "Mokola virus" right on the first page. Now you can try your hand at eMedicine, PubMed or any other trustworthy sites like that of the CDC and WHO to find more about these conditions.

Instead of a manual search, an appropriately designed CDSS could present these queries (with answers and further hyperlinks) in a systematic manner and retrieve the best possible queries required for approaching such a case. When married to an Electronic Medical Record with Internet capability, the CDSS could even make use of specific clinical data residing in the EMR. It can be seen that CDSS and Internet resources are complementary in nature – the latter is covered in greater detail in Chapter 6.

Conclusions and Future Directions

Because of the daily advent of new treatment modalities, decision making in patient care becomes increasingly complex. Often, a large amount of information has to be processed, much of which is quantifiable. Intuitive thought process involves rapid unconscious data processing and combines available information by law of average and, therefore, has a low intra- and inter-person consistency. So, the clinician of today should move towards analytic decision-making which, albeit typically slow, consciously, consistently and clearly spells out the basis for decision making.

Computerized diagnostics (including searching appropriate evidence) and clinical acumen are not mutually exclusive; rather they should reinforce each other for optimizing clinical care and patient outcomes. However, despite sophisticated gadgetry gaining the upper hand in many sectors of medical practice, the "human touch" should not be overlooked or forgotten.

As Pradhan[20] aptly sums up: "The good news is that we have the technology to deal with these problems. All pieces exist today: Evidence-based decision support systems, advanced techniques in research synthesis, alerting systems for clinical risk management, secure transactions for electronic data interchange, handheld computers and wireless networking. The good news is that we do not need to wait for breakthroughs in information technology or statistics to deal with challenges of today's healthcare system – most of the requisite theory and technology exist today. The bad news is that the barriers to progress are much harder than making technological breakthroughs. The barriers lie in changing people, and in changing systems: they lie in changing the culture of healthcare organizations, they lie in enlightening politicians and high-level bureaucrats, they lie in changing the funding authorities' view of research, and the barriers lie in the form of corporate ownership of information."

A major goal in years to come should be to raise the awareness of all healthcare delivery professionals so that the use (and building) of innovative and practically grounded evidence-based decision support systems are encouraged and fostered.

References

1. Sackett DL, Straus SE, Richardson WS, Rosenberg W, Haynes RB. *Evidence-based Medicine: How to Practice and Teach EBM*. 2nd ed. New York, NY: Churchill Livingstone; 2000.
2. Mendelson D, Carino TV. Evidence-based medicine. In: The United States—de rigueur or dream deferred? *Health Affairs*. 2005; 24: 133-136. doi: 10.1377/hlthaff.24.1.133.
3. Hersh W. Medical informatics education: an alternative pathway for training informationists. *J Med Libr Assoc*. 2002, 90(1): 76-79.
4. Shearer BS, Seymour A, Capitani C. Bringing the best of medical librarianship to the patient team. *J Med Libr Assoc*. 2001; 90: 22-31.
5. Sarbadhikari SN. "Medical informatics — are the doctors ready?" (Guest Editorial). *J. Indian Med. Assoc*. 1995, 93: 165-166.
6. Sarbadhikari SN. Basic medical education must include medical informatics. *Indian J Physiol. Pharamcol*. 2004a; 48(4): 395-408.
7. Sarbadhikari, SN. Automated diagnostic systems. *Indian Journal of Medical Informatics*. 2004b; 1: 25-28. [Also accessible at http://open-med.nic.in/218/]
8. Schwartz A, Millam G. A web-based library consult service for evidence-based medicine: technical development. *BMC Medical Informatics and Decision Making*. 2006; 6:16 doi: 10.1186/1472-6947-6-16 http://www.biomedcentral.com/1472-6947/6/16
9. Sotos G, MYCIN and NEOMYCIN: two approaches to generating explanations in rule-based expert systems. *Aviat Space Environ Med*. 1990; 61: 950-954.
10. de Dombal FT. Computer-aided diagnosis and medical decision support are not synonymous. *Methods Inf Med*. 1995; 34: 369-370.
11. Lemaire JB, et al. Effectiveness of the quick medical reference as a diagnostic tool. CMAJ. September 21, 1999; 161 (6) http://www.cmaj.ca/cgi/content/full/161/6/725
12. Berner ES, et al. Performance of four computer-based diagnostic systems. *N Engl J Med*. 1994; 330: 1792-1796.
13. Bergman LG, Fors UG. Computer-aided DSM-IV-diagnostics – acceptance, use and perceived usefulness in relation to users' learning styles. *BMC Med Inform Decis Mak*. 2005; 5:1.
14. Tan K, Dear PR, Newell SJ. Clinical decision support systems for neonatal care. *Cochrane Database Syst Rev*. 2005; 2: CD004211.
15. Garg AX, et al. Effects of computerized clinical decision support systems on practitioner performance and patient outcomes: a systematic review. *JAMA*. 2005; 293:1223-38.

16. Sim I, Gorman P, Greenes RA, Haynes RB, Kaplan B, Lehmann H, Tang PC. Clinical decision support systems for the practice of evidence-based medicine. *J Am Med Inform Assoc.* 2001; 8:527-534.
17. Haynes RB. Of studies, syntheses, synopses, and systems: the "4S" evolution of services for finding current best evidence. *Evidence-Based Medicine.* 2001; 6:36-38. http://ebm.bmjjournals.com/cgi/reprint/6/2/36
18. Kunnamo I, et al. 2005, National Decision support database based on computer-readable guidelines and using structured data from electronic patient records
http://www.terveysportti.fi/pls/kotisivut/docs/f1917377807/ gin_poster_decision_support_v2.pdf (Accessed July 2006)
19. Steinberg EP, Luce BR. Evidence based? caveat emptor! Health Affairs. 2005; 24: 80-92. doi: 10.1377/hlthaff.24.1.80
20. Pradhan M. The crystal ball - the future of informatics and decision making. http://www.informatics.adelaide.edu.au/topics/DS/MP-CrystalBall Talk.html. 2001 (Accessed July 2006)

Recommended Resources

Useful websites

1. Sarbadhikari SN. A CDSS for diagnosing amenorrhea. www.geocities. com/ drsupten. 2007.
2. Smith S. The classification algorithm. http://www.cs.mdx.ac.uk/ staff-pages/ serengul/The.Classification.algorithm.htm (Accessed July 2006).
3. http://www.ebm-guidelines.com

Articles

1. de Lusignan S, Lakhani M, Chan T. The role of informatics in continuing professional development quality improvement in primary care. *J Postgrad Med.* 2003, 49: 163-165.
2. Kavitha S, Sarbadhikari SN, Rao Ananth N. Implementation of decision tree classifier using classification algorithm for some inborn errors of metabolism. *Proc. Global Convention and Exposition on Telemedicine and eHealth.* New Delhi, 17-22 August, 2006.
3. Master-Hunter T, Heiman DL. Amenorrhea: evaluation and treatment. *American Family Physician.* 2006, 73: 1374-1382 http://www.aafp.org/ afp/20060415/1374.html
4. Sarbadhikari SN. The state of medical informatics in India: a roadmap for optimal organization. *J. Medical Systems.* 2005; 29: 125-141.

Index

Accuracy, 2, 3, 77, 113, 114, 116, 117, 118, 119, 120, 121, 123, 124, 125, 128, 131, 132, 138
Alternative hypothesis, 31, 46, 47, 48
ANOVA, 52-54

B

Bar graph, 35
Bayesian analysis, 121, 126, 170
Belmont report, 8
Bias, 64
Bimodal distribution, 38
Binomial, 43, 50
Bioengineering, 143
Bioethics, 18, 27
Biosis, 88
Biostatistical tools, 28-29
Biostatistics, 4, 28-60, 107, 108, 136, 138
Blinding, 104, 106, 108, 115, 116
Boolean operators, 88

C

Case-control study, see retrospective studies

Case reports, 66-67
Case series, 66-67
Categorical variables, 51, 52
Causality, 65-66
CBR, 170
CDSS, 3, 5, 166-177
Censoring, 58
Chance, 46, 47, 55, 65, 73, 80, 94, 97, 99, 109, 112, 126, 152, 169
Classification of variables, 29-31
Clinical trial, 2, 26, 43, 116, 118, 143, 146
Cochrane databse, 84-85, 92, 167, 171, 176
Cohort studies, see prospective studies
Confidence intervals, 45-46, 108, 146, 151
COPE guidelines, 12, 17-27
Correlation, 40-42, 59, 113, 123, 128
Cost-effectiveness analysis, 73-74
Covariance, 59
Cox regression model, 58
Critical appraisal, 96-101

D

Database, 84, 85, 86, 87, 88, 89, 172, 173, 177
Data collection, 28, 33-34
Decision making, 74, 76, 77, 78, 82, 130, 141, 173, 175, 177
Declaration of Helsinki, 10
Descriptive data analysis, 37-44
Dispersion, 38

E

EBM, 1, 4-6, 89
    diagnosis and, 111-133
    economic analysis and, 141-158
    medical informatics and, 166-177
    overview, 93-103
    prognosis and, 134-140
    therapy and, 104-110
    translating into practice, 159-165
Efficacy, 10, 31, 46, 116, 128, 129, 131, 132, 173
EMBase, 88
EMR, 3, 4, 5, 63, 160, 175
Epidemiology, 4, 93, 95, 132, 163
Ethics, 4, 7-27, 68, 98
Evidence pyramid, 83-84
Expert system, 172-173

F

Frequency, 34, 35, 38, 135
Fryback/Thornbury
    hierarchy, 128-29

G

Good clinical practice (GCP), 10

H

Health related quality of life (HRQoL), 135
Histogram, 34-35
Hypothesis, 9, 21, 29, 31, 32, 105
Hypothesis testing, 46-54

I

Incidence, 77, 107, 143, 151, 156
Incremental cost-effectiveness ratio (ICER), 143
Inferential testing, 44-54
Informatics, 2, 3, 5, 166, 167, 168, 169, 174, 176, 177
Interquartile range, 39
Intervention, 32, 63, 68, 69, 79, 81, 95, 99, 100, 105, 106, 107, 108, 109, 113, 134, 135, 137, 139, 142, 143, 146, 147, 152, 153, 155, 171, 173

K

Kaplan-Meier curve, 58
Kappa statistic, 65
Kruskal-Wallis test, 54
Kurtosis, 40

L

Likelihood ratio, 57
Line graph, 36

M

MANCOVA, 59
MANOVA, 59
Mean, 37, 39, 40, 43, 44, 45, 46, 47, 48, 49, 100, 109, 123, 144, 151, 170
Measures of central tendency, 37-38

Measures of dispersion, 38-39
Median, 37, 40, 43, 171
MESH headings, 87-88
Mesokurtic, 40
Meta-analysis, 59-60
Mode, 37, 38, 40, 43, 170
Modeling, 146, 156
Multivariate analysis, 59

N

Normal distribution, 43
Null hypothesis, 31, 47

O

Odds ratio, 57
Opportunity cost, 146-147
Outcome, 29, 42, 64, 74, 78, 81, 88,
 95, 97, 99, 100, 105, 107, 108,
 109, 111, 113, 118, 129, 135,
 137, 138, 153, 171
Outliers, 37

P

PACS, 3
Parametric tests, 53
Pie chart, 35-36
Plagiarism, 12, 17, 26
Poisson distribution, 43
Population, 2, 28, 29, 32, 37, 45, 46,
 47, 48, 49, 50, 51, 53, 55, 75,
 76, 77, 80, 81, 95, 97, 117, 119,
 121, 123, 125, 136, 141, 148,
 158
Power, 18, 31, 32, 97, 99, 118, 162
Precision, 77, 85, 113, 139
Prediction, 42
Predictive values, 55, 56, 77, 88,
 111, 124, 125
Prevalence, 55, 56, 78, 98, 117,
 121, 124, 125, 126

Probability, 31, 32, 42, 45, 47, 55,
 56, 57, 77, 78, 80, 81, 99, 111,
 113, 117, 121, 124, 125, 126,
 127, 128, 129, 150, 173
Proportion, 35, 47, 50, 51, 76, 77,
 118, 138, 147, 170
Prospective studies, 67-68,
PubMed, 86-88, 90, 91, 95, 103,
 162, 165, 169, 174
PubMedCentral, 103, 165

Q

QALY, 154-155
Qualitative data, 29, 30, 38, 111
Quantitative data, 29, 30, 38, 72, 81,
 111
Quartiles, 39
Questionnaire, 33, 63, 67

R

Randomization, 68, 104, 105, 106,
 108, 116
Randomized controlled trial, 68
Range, 38
Regression analysis, 42, 59
Relative risk, 56
Reliability, 61, 65
Research, 1, 2, 7, 8, 12, 15, 18, 27,
 28, 29, 61, 63, 64, 66, 69, 70,
 83, 89, 92, 131
Research design, 66-68
Research methodology, 61-71
Retrospective studies, 67, 70, 104-
 105, 114-116, 136
Risk, 9, 31, 56, 57, 62, 66, 69, 80,
 82, 87, 88, 95, 98, 104, 105,
 106, 107, 108, 112, 116, 118,
 119, 120, 125, 130, 134, 136,
 139, 147, 148, 149, 150, 154,
 155, 156, 173, 174, 175

Risk reduction,
  absolute, 108
  relative, 108
ROC curve, 56, 123, 124, 129

S

Sample size, 32, 33, 45, 47, 48, 49,
  50, 60, 63, 99, 106
SAS, 57
Scatter diagram, 41-42
Sensitivity, 54-56, 76, 87, 121-123,
  126, 127, 129, 132, 155
Significance, 31, 47, 61, 66
Simulation, 81, 147
Skewness, 39
Sources of evidence, 83-92
Spearman's co-efficient, 41
Specificity, 54-56, 76, 121-123, 126,
  127, 129
SPSS, 48, 57
Standard deviation, 39
Statistical significance, 66, 99

STATA, 57
Study design, 96-98
SUMsearch, 89
Survival analysis, 58-59
Systematic sampling, 32

T

TRIP database, 89
Tuskeegee study, 8

U

Uncertainty, 75-78

V

Validity, 9, 11, 32, 65, 75, 77, 91, 96,
  97, 98, 99, 107, 112, 113, 115,
  116, 119, 120, 137, 138
Variance, 39

W

Wilcoxon test, 54